HOW TO

OUTSMART

YOUR

ALLERGIES

Art Ulene, MD

in collaboration with

The Asthma & Allergy Foundation of America

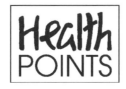

This book has been written and published strictly for informational purposes, and in no way should it be used as a substitute for consultation with your medical doctor or healthcare professional. You should not consider educational material herein to be the practice of medicine or to replace consultation with a physician or other medical practitioner. The author and publisher urge all readers to be aware of their health status and to consult health professionals before beginning any health or fitness program, including changes in dietary habits and physical activity.

Published by: HealthPOINTS

Feeling Fine Company LLC

13160 Mindanao Way, Suite 270

Marina del Rey, CA 90292

Designed by: Media Content Marketing

405 Park Avenue, Suite 901

New York, NY 10022

Cover Design by: Lee Meyers

ISBN: 0-932513-23-9

Printed in the USA

HOW TO

OUTSMART

YOUR

ALLERGIES

Acknowledgments

The author gratefully acknowledges the contributions of the following individuals:

- The allergy experts who willingly offered suggestions and reviewed the material:

  John Anderson, MD
  Linda Borschuk
  Steven Brunton, MD
  Peter Creticos, MD
  Mary Lou Hayden, RN, MS, C-FNP
  Margaret Heagarty, MD
  Robert Lanier, MD
  Phillip Lieberman, MD
  Floyd Malveaux, MD
  Harold S. Nelson, MD
  Gary Rachelefsky, MD
  Martin Weisberg, MD

- The Asthma & Allergy Foundation of America, especially Linda Sorin, MBA, Mary Worstell, MPH and Sharon Hipkins, MSN, RN for their efforts and support.
- Richard Trubo, Gretchen Henkel, Valerie Ulene, MD and Laura Bellotti for their research, writing and editing skills.
- Donna Pepe, Communications Strategies, Inc., for her enthusiastic support.
- Kukla Vera, Jean Drummond and Jamie McDowell for their talents and tireless efforts.

*This edition of **How To Outsmart Your Allergies** has been made available by Schering Corporation.*

Table of Contents

Introduction

Recent research has given us a much clearer understanding of allergies, and this has resulted in vastly improved prevention strategies and treatments. Thanks to these scientific advances, most allergic persons are now able to lead completely normal lives—free of the physical discomfort and social inconvenience that allergies can produce.

Nevertheless, millions of Americans continue to suffer from allergy symptoms. About one out of every 11 office visits to a physician is for an allergic disease, and allergic rhinitis (also known as "hay fever") is the single most common chronic human disease, accounting for one out of every 40 visits to doctors' offices.

Many people (and some physicians) treat allergies as nothing more than a minor inconvenience, and in some cases that may be appropriate. But allergic symptoms can also be disabling—decreasing productivity at work, interfering with school attendance, spoiling recreational activities and complicating social relationships. In severe cases, allergies can lead to serious, even potentially life-threatening, conditions such as asthma.

Many people suffer needlessly because they simply don't realize that their symptoms—including their asthma symptoms—may be caused or triggered by allergies. Others know they are allergic but have not learned how to manage their problem correctly. They remain in contact with the allergens that trigger their reactions, and they treat themselves inappropriately. As a result, their symptoms persist, or even worsen.

But *you* don't have to suffer. There are many ways to overcome the problems that allergies can cause, and you will read about them in this book. We'll show you how to identify the specific allergens that trigger your allergic reactions and how to avoid—or at least minimize—further contact with them. You will learn which medications you can use when it's not possible to completely avoid your allergy triggers, and we'll describe *when* and *how* to use these drugs for maximum effectiveness.

Armed with this information, you can take a much more active—and more effective—role in the management of your allergies. You'll also be much better prepared to work with your doctor if your self-care strategies do not provide enough relief from your symptoms.

No matter what your past experience with allergies has been, it's important to know that you don't have to suffer any longer from allergy symptoms. Using the information in this book, and working in partnership with your physician, you should soon be able to enjoy the relief that modern science has made possible.

We wish you success in this endeavor, and good health always.

Art Ulene, MD
and
The Asthma & Allergy
Foundation of America

Chapter I

What is an Allergy?

An allergy is an inappropriate reaction by your immune system. The job of the immune system is to identify harmful foreign substances, such as viruses and bacteria, and get rid of them before they can make you sick. The immune system does this by creating antibodies to combat these foreign invaders.

In people with allergies, however, the immune system is overly sensitive. It reacts inappropriately by producing antibodies against *harmless* substances, called allergens, such as pollens, mold spores, animal dander, dust mites, or even foods or drugs. In a nonallergic person, contact with these allergens will not normally cause an allergic reaction, although some of them might be irritating to the body in other ways.

Why does the immune system overreact to everyday substances this way? The answer revolves around special antibodies called IgE (immunoglobulin E), which are key players in an allergic reaction. Scientists believe that these so-called antibodies are "left over" from prehistoric times when they were needed to help destroy or contain parasitic infections. Everyone *makes* or *produces* IgE, but allergic individuals have inherited the tendency to make *large* quantities of it in response to one or more substances that are inappropriately recognized by the immune system as being "foreign." This excessive production of special antibodies triggers the release of chemicals that can cause the physical changes and symptoms associated with allergies: itchy nose, eyes and skin; repeated sneezing, nasal congestion and coughing; dark circles under the eyes; throat or palate itching; or frequent throat clearing. However, in some people, allergic reactions can actually reach life-threatening proportions.

ALLERGIES AND HEREDITY

Allergies tend to run in families. Your own risk of developing allergies is strongly related to your parents' allergy history. If neither parent is allergic, your risk of developing allergies is about 15-25%. If one parent is allergic, your risk is about 30-50%. If both parents are allergic, your risk is about 60-75%.

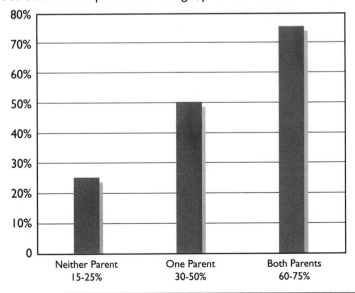

COMMON AIRBORNE ALLERGENS (AEROALLERGENS)

Pollens (trees, grasses, weeds)

Mold and mildew spores

Dust mites and their debris (decaying body parts, fecal waste)

Animal dander and saliva (fur or feathered animals)

Animal urinary protein

Cockroaches and their debris (decaying body parts, fecal matter, saliva)

OTHER PREVALENT ALLERGENS

Venom from stinging insects (bees, yellow jackets, hornets, wasps, fire ants)

Drug proteins (such as penicillin)

Latex

Food proteins (such as milk, eggs, peanuts)

Occupational chemicals

Although no one is *born* with allergies, you can *inherit the tendency* to develop them. However, you may not have the same allergies as your parents. For example, you may be allergic to mold, while your mother is allergic to dust mites. Or you might be allergic to an airborne allergen (such as pollen), whereas your brother is allergic to a food protein (such as from peanuts). We still are not sure what determines *which* substances a person with allergic tendencies will ultimately react to. But we do know that you must be personally exposed to a particular substance before you can become allergic to it. Studies also show that the more often and more directly you come in contact with an allergen, the more likely you are to develop an allergy to it.

Allergies usually begin in childhood, although they can show up at any age. The most common allergic problems among infants are food allergies and eczema (patches of dry, itchy skin). In older children, allergic rhinitis ("hay fever") is more common. As some children get older, their symptoms decline, only to reappear later in life. Why this happens in some people and not in others remains a mystery.

The Most Common Allergic Reactions

There are several common allergy disorders. Although they may appear significantly different from one another, all share the same basic underlying processes. The following brief descriptions will introduce you to these disorders, which you will find described in more detail later in this book.

Allergic rhinitis (or "hay fever") is an inflammation of the mucous membranes in the nose that occurs after an allergen is inhaled. The inflammation can also involve membranes in the sinuses and ear passages. Common symptoms and signs include:

- nasal stuffiness
- sneezing
- nasal itching
- runny nose
- itching of the ears
- itching of the roof of the mouth
- postnasal drainage ("drip")

In some people, allergic rhinitis occurs only at particular times of the year—usually when local plants are pollinating or during prolonged periods of high humidity, when mold spore levels are high. These individuals are said to have *seasonal* allergic rhinitis.

Others experience allergic symptoms throughout the year, a condition known as *perennial* allergic rhinitis. In this group, the offending allergens are more likely to come from dust mites, cockroaches and pets. However, in warmer areas like Southern California and Florida, pollen can also cause *perennial* (or practically year-round) problems.

Allergic conjunctivitis is an inflammation of the delicate transparent tissues that cover the white portion of the eyeball and the underside of the eyelids. Common symptoms and signs include:
 • redness over the eyeball and underside of the eyelids
 • watering of the eyes
 • itching around the eyes
 • puffiness of the surrounding eye tissue

Allergic conjunctivitis may occur seasonally or perennially, depending on which allergens are triggering the reaction and how often an individual is exposed to them.

Atopic dermatitis (eczema) is a skin condition that commonly causes the following symptoms and signs:
 • itching, redness and dryness of the skin, usually in the elbow creases, behind the knees, on the back of the neck and around the eyes (in children, symptoms may first appear on the face, then spread to the chest, arms and legs).

Atopic dermatitis can occur at any time of the year. It is often triggered by allergic reactions to certain foods (such as fish, eggs, wheat or peanuts). Exposure to dust mites can cause the condition, too.

Urticaria (hives) is a skin lesion that can appear on any part of the body. Hives can be the result of an allergic reaction (allergens in foods and drugs are the most common causes) or they can have a nonallergic origin (for example, a viral infection, physical pressure or exposure to cold air). Often no cause is evident. Common symptoms and signs of hives include:

- raised, red welts
- itching

Asthma is a respiratory disorder that is triggered, in many cases, by allergies. When people with asthma are exposed to particular allergens, they may develop signs and symptoms such as:

- chest tightness
- shortness of breath
- coughing
- wheezing

Anaphylaxis is a life-threatening allergic reaction that affects many organs throughout the body at the same time. The symptoms usually occur within moments of exposure to the offending allergen, and can include:

- flushing
- a red, itchy rash (urticaria)
- swelling and congestion of the nose, tongue and throat
- swelling of the soft tissue under the skin (angioedema)
- nausea and vomiting
- wheezing and shortness of breath
- decline in blood pressure

What Occurs in an Allergic Reaction?

A lot happens when you are exposed to an allergen. Several steps must occur before you'll experience allergic symptoms such as a runny nose or sneezing. Each of these steps is a point at which an intervention can take place (with medications, for example) to prevent or ease these symptoms.

Here is how an allergic reaction unfolds:

- For an allergic reaction to occur, you must first become *sensitized* to the responsible allergen. In your initial encounter with pollen, for example, even though you won't have any noticeable allergic symptoms, your body may become sensitized to allergenic protein from the pollen. As you inhale the pollen particles, your body will form IgE antibodies that position themselves on the surface of certain cells—called mast cells and basophils—that line the respiratory tract (nasal tissue and breathing tubes). Although these allergy-causing cells are present in all tissues in the body, they are most prevalent in tissues of the skin, the nasal lining, the lungs and the digestive tract. Nothing bad happens after this first exposure to the allergen, but the attachment of IgE antibodies to these cells sensitizes the immune system and sets the stage for subsequent allergy symptoms.

- Next, during subsequent exposures to pollen, certain cells in the nose will respond to the allergenic protein from the pollen grain. As this protein comes in contact with mast cells and basophils, it will interact with IgE antibodies as though there were a lock-and-key arrangement. As this happens, the mast cells or basophils become "turned on," and release chemicals such as histamine, which create the classic signs and symptoms of allergies. Histamine plays no favorites where it does its work. For example:
  — When histamine comes in contact with nerve endings, it causes sneezing and itching.

— When it comes in contact with mucus-secreting glands, it increases their production of mucus.

— When it comes in contact with small blood vessels, it causes leakage of fluid from the vessels and nasal congestion.

At the same time, other chemicals (such as prostaglandins and leukotrienes in the mast cells and basophils) are released and act on the same glands and blood vessels. As this happens, other symptoms can develop or existing symptoms—including nasal congestion and nasal secretions—may worsen, thus adding to the evolving problem.

• As these acute events are occurring, another insidious process is unfolding at sites like the nasal mucosa and other areas exposed to the external world. Some of the allergen is being "picked up" by a special cell, called an antigen-presenting cell (or APC), which brings the allergen into contact with other types of cells called T-cells. When this happens, the T-cells release a variety of chemicals of their own, which in turn trigger a process that produces even more IgE antibodies. It's a complicated process. But the result may be quite familiar: a further fueling of the allergic reaction.

When people suffer from allergic rhinitis, their symptoms may surface and make them miserable each time they cut the grass or play with a cat. But when they're exposed to grass pollen over the entire course of the grass pollen season, something more can happen: They are apt to develop *chronic, persistent* symptoms, caused by the frequent release of inflammatory chemicals into the nasal tissues and the resulting intense inflammatory process. So they not only will experience acute symptoms each time they mow the lawn,

WHAT ABOUT ASTHMA?

This is a book about allergies, but we will devote a chapter (Chapter 11) to the topic of asthma. That's because asthma is a complex disorder that often has allergies as its basis; in fact, allergy is the "driving force" for asthmatic episodes in many patients with this condition. Even though multiple factors are capable of inducing asthma, research shows that allergens can reach the lower airways and trigger an allergic asthmatic response.

You might be playing with a cat, for example, and start to experience acute symptoms such as chest tightness, shortness of breath, coughing and/or wheezing; these symptoms are reflective of mast cell activity leading to inflammation. If you're exposed to a cat chronically (perhaps it sleeps in your bed), a process involving T-cells unfolds, attracting cells such as eosinophils and basophils into the lungs, producing chronic, persistent asthma. An ongoing inflammatory process underlies this chronic form of asthma, and once your airways are primed, daily exposure to allergens can cause a persistent, insidious reaction with chronic asthmatic symptoms. Also, as with pure allergies, the sensitization of the lower airways can produce a "hyperirritable" state that, in the presence of irritants (such as pollution and cigarette smoke) or other factors (weather changes, exercise, viral infections), can produce symptoms.

but more significantly, they'll develop chronic symptoms that persist throughout the grass pollen season—10 to 20 weeks in duration.

Another complicating factor is the development of "non-specific reactivity," which means that as the airways become sensitized, they may react not just to pollen, for example, but to a variety of irritants—air pollution, cigarette smoke, perfume and hair spray, among others.

These irritants do not cause true allergic reactions (in other words, they do not involve the immune system and IgE antibodies), but they can directly, physically irritate sensitive noses, eyes and airways, and the resulting symptoms may feel just as uncomfortable as a real allergic reaction. Non-specific reactivity can occur by itself or after the tissues become chronically inflamed.

The Source of Your Own Allergies

Allergic reactions most commonly affect the upper and lower respiratory tract, gastrointestinal tract and/or skin, because these are the organs where the greatest concentrations of mast cells are found. The spectrum of symptoms can vary, influenced by the site at which your body comes in contact with the allergen:

- **You can inhale allergens.** Many potential allergens are carried in the air we breathe. This puts the allergens in contact with immune cells located in tissues that line the nose, mouth, throat, trachea and breathing passages of the lungs. Examples of commonly inhaled allergens include plant pollens and mold spores; airborne animal dander, saliva and urine; and particles from dust mites and cockroaches and their waste. Inhaled allergens are more likely to cause symptoms related to the respiratory tract, such as a runny nose, sneezing, itchy eyes or nose, nasal congestion, sinus pressure, postnasal drip, cough, chest tightness and wheezing.

- **You can ingest allergens.** Some allergens are contained in the substances we swallow. This puts them in contact with immune cells located in the lining of the gastrointestinal tract. Examples of commonly ingested allergens include foods such as eggs, milk, nuts and seafood; and drugs such as penicillin and sulfa. Ingested

THE ALLERGIC PROCESS: What Happens in a Nonallergic Person

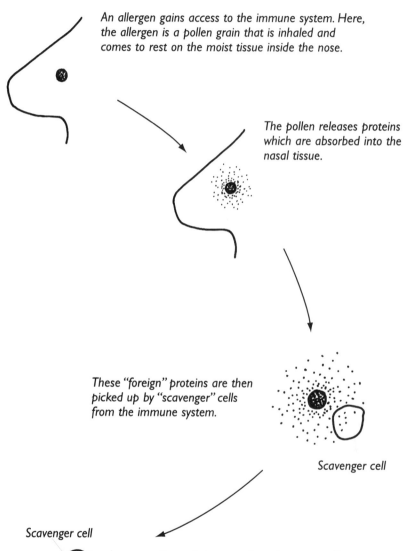

An allergen gains access to the immune system. Here, the allergen is a pollen grain that is inhaled and comes to rest on the moist tissue inside the nose.

The pollen releases proteins which are absorbed into the nasal tissue.

These "foreign" proteins are then picked up by "scavenger" cells from the immune system.

Scavenger cell

Scavenger cell

In a nonallergenic person, these immune cells dispose of the foreign proteins, and the process ends.

THE ALLERGIC PROCESS: What Happens in an Allergic Person After the First Exposure to an Allergen

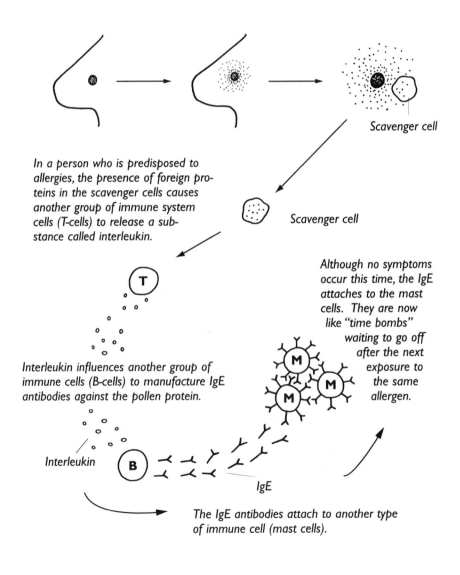

Scavenger cell

In a person who is predisposed to allergies, the presence of foreign proteins in the scavenger cells causes another group of immune system cells (T-cells) to release a substance called interleukin.

Scavenger cell

Although no symptoms occur this time, the IgE attaches to the mast cells. They are now like "time bombs" waiting to go off after the next exposure to the same allergen.

Interleukin influences another group of immune cells (B-cells) to manufacture IgE antibodies against the pollen protein.

Interleukin

IgE

The IgE antibodies attach to another type of immune cell (mast cells).

THE ALLERGIC PROCESS: What Happens in an Allergic Person After Sensitization Has Occurred

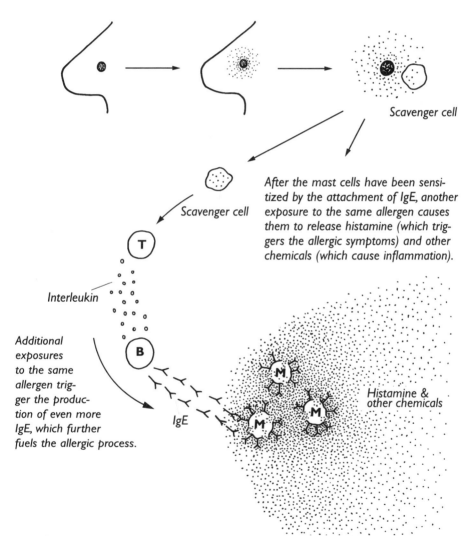

Scavenger cell

Scavenger cell

T

After the mast cells have been sensitized by the attachment of IgE, another exposure to the same allergen causes them to release histamine (which triggers the allergic symptoms) and other chemicals (which cause inflammation).

Interleukin

Additional exposures to the same allergen trigger the production of even more IgE, which further fuels the allergic process.

B

IgE

Histamine & other chemicals

If a person is exposed to the same allergen continuously—as often happens during pollen season—a persistent form of inflammation may develop. This can cause symptoms to persist long after exposure to the allergen has stopped.

allergens are more likely to cause skin manifestations and, to a lesser degree, gastrointestinal symptoms, including abdominal pain, cramps, bloody diarrhea, nausea and vomiting. If the reaction to an ingested allergen becomes severe, the symptoms may be more generalized with swelling, hives or even "shock" (reflecting a drop in blood pressure).

- **You can contact allergens via your skin.** You might be licked by a cat, roll in the grass, or touch poison ivy or oak—any of which can create an allergic skin response. Doctors use the term "contact dermatitis" to describe the itchy rash that occurs when the skin comes in contact with substances such as poison ivy.

- **Allergens can be injected into your body.** Many potential allergens are injected directly into the body through insect stings or medical procedures. This route of access rapidly puts the allergens into the bloodstream, spreading them to other sites throughout the body (this is one reason why allergic reactions to injected allergens can be so severe). Examples of commonly injected allergens include venom from flying insects, such as honey and bumblebees, wasps, yellow jackets and hornets, and medications administered intramuscularly or intravenously. Injected allergens are most likely to cause local redness, swelling and pain, but they can also cause rashes all over the body and life-threatening anaphylactic reactions that require immediate attention to prevent death.

In spite of this general tendency for allergic symptoms to reflect the way your body came in contact with the allergen, there is no hard and fast rule about this. For example, allergic skin rashes can occur as a result of ingesting a food to which you are allergic.

What determines the severity of your allergic reaction? It is generally related to the intensity of the exposure (the amount of allergen to which you are exposed). However, some people are so sensitive to certain allergens that even miniscule doses of the allergen can trigger life-threatening reactions. This severe type of reaction ("anaphylaxis") can occur in response to a bee sting, to ingesting a particular food or to receiving a drug, for example. If you've ever had a severe allergic reaction, you should do everything possible to avoid any further exposure to the offending substance, and you may need to carry lifesaving medications, such as adrenaline (epinephrine), with you in case of an inadvertent or accidental exposure that could cause another severe reaction.

Keep in mind that allergic reactions may be site-specific (confined to the nose, chest, skin or abdomen, for example); in these cases, "localized" mast cells, such as those in the nose, are producing the response. Or reactions may be more generalized, and a number of different body systems may be involved; in these cases, a more generalized mast cell process is occurring throughout the body, as allergens are exposed to these mast cells at many different sites. For example, if you are stung by a bee, the allergen is not only deposited at the site of the injection, but some of it gets into the bloodstream and is carried throughout the body.

Summary

An allergy is an inappropriate reaction by your immune system to a normally harmless substance. These substances, called allergens, can be inhaled (aeroallergens), ingested (foods) or injected (drugs, venoms). The aeroallergens are substances that you may encounter every day. They include plant pollens, molds, pets (dander, saliva, urine), dust mites (body parts, fecal material) and insects (body parts, fecal material, saliva).

Irritating substances can compound the problem of an already inflamed airway in an allergic patient. These irritants include air pollution, industrial chemicals, perfumes, aerosols and cleaning products.

Allergies can be disruptive, but you can learn to manage them through self-help measures and proper medication. The rest of this book will show you how.

Chapter 2

Outdoor Allergens

If allergy symptoms send you running for cover whenever you step outdoors, you are probably reacting to either pollens or mold spores in the air. These two categories of allergens are the most common causes of itchy, watery eyes, runny nose, sneezing and nasal congestion in a patient who suffers from seasonal allergic rhinitis ("hay fever"). Proteins from these sources can even find their way to the lungs to trigger asthma. It is estimated that about 35 million Americans are allergic to these airborne allergens, and the problem is not limited to the outdoors. Airborne pollen and mold can sneak into your home through open windows and doors and on your clothing and hair, or on the fur of pets. When this happens, the same symptoms can occur indoors.

In most people, reactions to these allergens tend to occur in seasonal patterns that correspond to the life cycles of plants. For example, tree pollens predominate in the early spring, so if you're allergic to them, this is the time of year when you're likely to experience symptoms. Grass pollens are most prevalent in the late spring through summer, while weed pollens cause problems in the spring through fall. In certain parts of the country, however, pollen can be almost a year-round allergen (for example, grass in Florida).

Molds have patterns of their own, and are most problematic during the fall, when leaves are decaying. Even so, molds can cause symptoms whenever conditions are damp or humid. In warm, humid climates, for example, molds can thrive outdoors throughout the year.

If you divide your time between different regions of the country, your allergy symptoms might seem to follow you. For instance, if you spend your summers in the north and travel south for the winter, you may experience symptoms throughout the year if you're allergic to the pollens or molds found in each location.

Since the most common symptoms triggered by outdoor allergens are sneezing, runny nose and nasal congestion, physicians refer to a seasonal pattern of symptoms as "seasonal allergic rhinitis" ("rhinitis" means inflammation of the tissues that line the nose). A more familiar name for this condition is "hay fever." The medical term for a year-round pattern of allergic symptoms is "*perennial* allergic rhinitis."

HAY FEVER: A MISNOMER

The term "hay fever" is commonly used to describe seasonal allergic rhinitis, but it is really a misnomer. This condition has nothing to do with hay, nor does it cause a fever. When British farmers and their doctors first coined the term in the 19th century, they erroneously concluded that springtime hay-cutting was causing congested sinuses, coughing, breathing difficulties and other symptoms. We now know, of course, that those symptoms are actually caused by plants that pollinate or molds that produce spores during the late springtime. Still, the term "hay fever" has lingered.

The best way to decrease your problems due to outdoor pollens and molds is to avoid all contact with them. Without actual contact with these allergens, you won't have reactions and you won't develop symptoms. Unfortunately, for many people, avoidance is often easier said than done. And, for some—like those who work outdoors—complete avoidance of pollens and molds is impossible.

Even if you cannot completely eliminate contact with these allergens, there are still many ways to decrease your exposure to them and minimize the impact they have on your life. You'll learn some of these techniques in the material that follows.

Pollens

After a long, cold winter, nothing could be more welcome than the first signs of spring—unless you suffer from pollen allergies. While your family and friends are enjoying the outdoors following months of blustery weather, your nose is plugging up, your eyes are red and watery, and you're sneezing or even wheezing. You don't need a doctor to tell you that pollen season has arrived.

Pollens are microscopic, round- or oval-shaped male reproductive plant cells that play an essential role in the plant fertilization process. Huge numbers of pollen granules are dispersed into the air by certain plants during their reproductive cycle. For example, a ragweed plant can release a million pollen grains in a single day.

Allergic reactions are triggered when the tiny granules are inhaled into the nose and come in contact with the nasal lining tissues. Allergenic substances are then released from the pollen and react with mast cells that have been previously sensitized. This causes the release of histamine and other chemicals into the lining tissues, which in turn causes the symptoms. The same reaction will occur and cause symptoms in the eyes and throat if pollen granules land on their surfaces.

Allergic rhinitis related to pollens (see maps and charts on pages 30-33) occurs most commonly in the spring and late summer, the times of year when allergenic plants produce most of their pollen. There is a very predictable pattern to the pollen release: In the first weeks of spring, trees like the elm, maple and birch release their pollen, followed by the ash, sycamore and oak; later in the spring and early summer, grass pollens spread into the air, often starting in early May and lasting through mid-July. Various weeds can begin to pollinate in the spring (such as sage) or summer (such as plantain). However, the dominant weeds (for example, ragweed) often produce their allergens in the late summer to fall, a process that may continue until the first frost.

As the regional allergen maps and charts indicate (see pages 30-33), pollen seasons vary from one part of the country to another. The

ARE YOUR ALLERGIES TRIGGERING ASTHMA?

Allergens such as pollen can trigger an allergic asthma episode in a suscep-tible individual. Although most pollen grains are too large to float freely into the lungs, much of the allergenic material in the air is much smaller. That's because, as millions of pollen grains fall to the ground, the problematic aller-genic protein is extracted from the pollen by moisture, dew or a light rain shower. This material is then suspended in the air on aerosol droplets or dust particles, which are so small (less than 10 microns in diameter) that they can easily make their way into the lungs to trigger asthma.

closer you live to the equator, the earlier the season starts. In fact, pollen can become problematic as early as January in the southern-most parts of the U.S.

Paying Attention to Pollen Counts

Many weather reports in newspapers and on television now include the airborne pollen counts in your community. These pollen reports are measurements of grains of pollen (usually per cubic meter of air), accumulated over a 24-hour period. Typically, these pollen grains are collected by trapping them on glass rods placed on rooftops; the number of grains are then counted under the microscope. The American Academy of Allergy, Asthma and Immunology (AAAAI) regularly reports pollen counts during the pollen season.

Pollen counts can help you decide when it's wise to remain indoors in air conditioning if you suffer from allergies. Bear in mind, however, that today's paper carries *yesterday's* readings. Today's counts may vary greatly if the weather changes significantly. Pollen counts tend to rise on dry, sunny and windy days, when pollen is more likely to be carried through the air and inhaled by simple breathing. Counts are also highest in the late morning and afternoon. However, pollen counts tend to be lower on overcast, rainy or non-breezy days.

How high do pollen counts need to be before they spell trouble? That varies from one person to another. Some individuals become symptomatic when counts are as low as 20 grains per cubic meter of air; but most allergy-prone people begin to sneeze and cough when the counts approach 100 (on a really "bad pollen day," the counts can reach 500). By tracking pollen counts and monitoring your symptoms, you'll get a sense of when conditions become problematic for you.

SOURCES OF OUTDOOR ALLERGENS

Here are many of the outdoor plants and trees that are sources of pollen in the U.S.:

GRASSES
Bahai
Bermuda
Bluegrass
Johnson
Orchard
Redtop
Sweet Vernal
Timothy

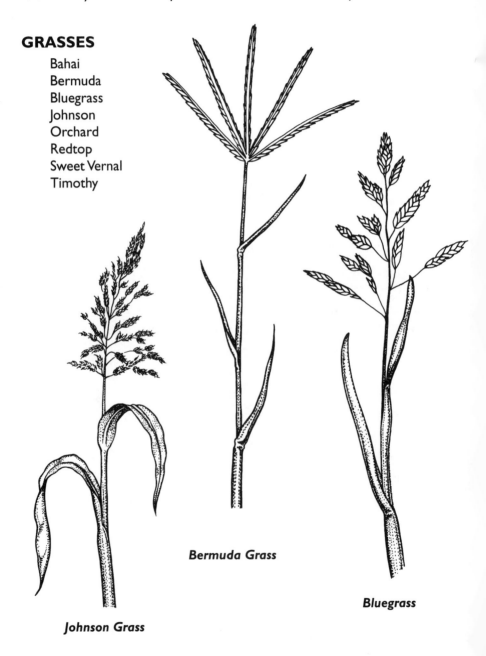

Bermuda Grass

Bluegrass

Johnson Grass

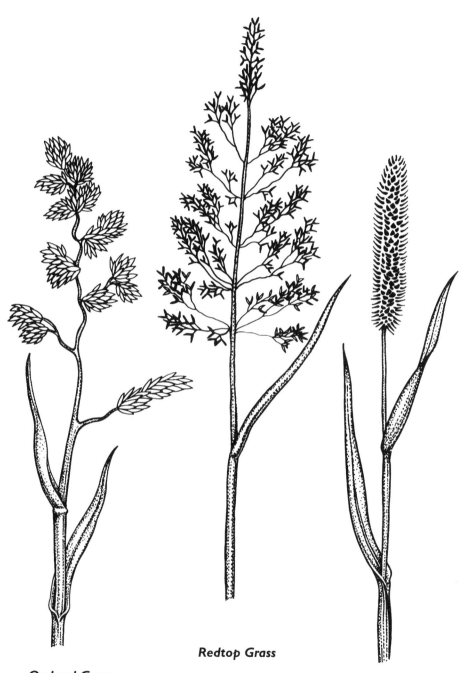

Orchard Grass

Redtop Grass

Timothy Grass

WEEDS

Burning Bush (Kochia)
Pigweed
Carelessweeds
Plantain
Cocklebur
Ragweed
Dock
Russian Thistle
Lamb's Quarter
Sagebrush

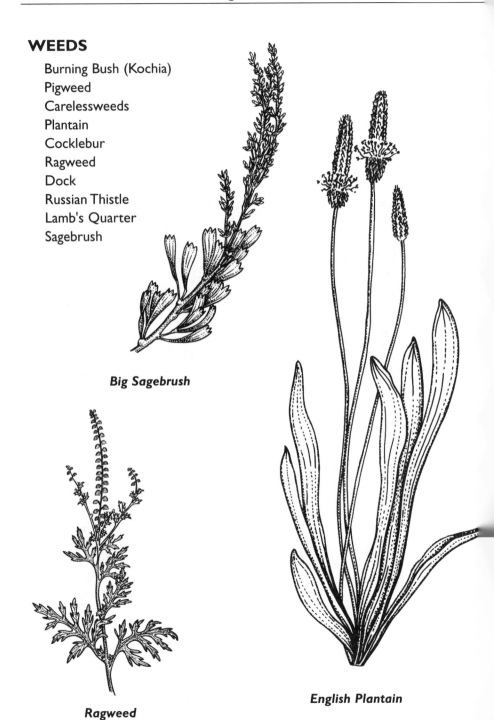

Big Sagebrush

Ragweed

English Plantain

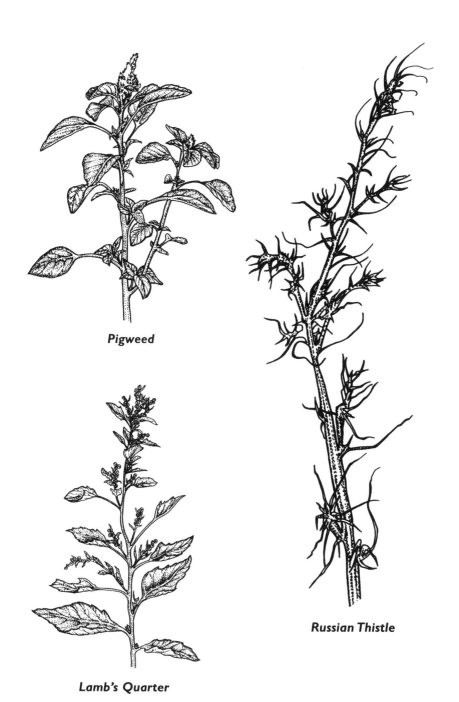

Pigweed

Lamb's Quarter

Russian Thistle

TREES

Alder family:
Alder
Birch

Ash family:
Ash
Olive
Privet

Juniper family:
Cedar
Juniper

Maple family:
Box Elder
Maple

Nut family:
Hickory
Pecan
Walnut

Oak family:
Beech
Oak

Poplar family:
Cottonwood
Poplar

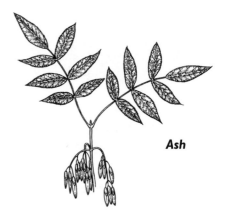

Ash

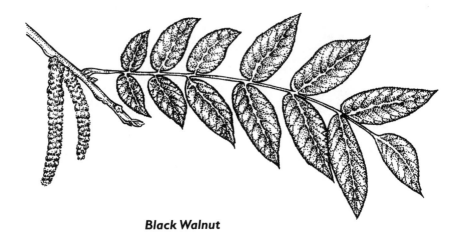

Black Walnut

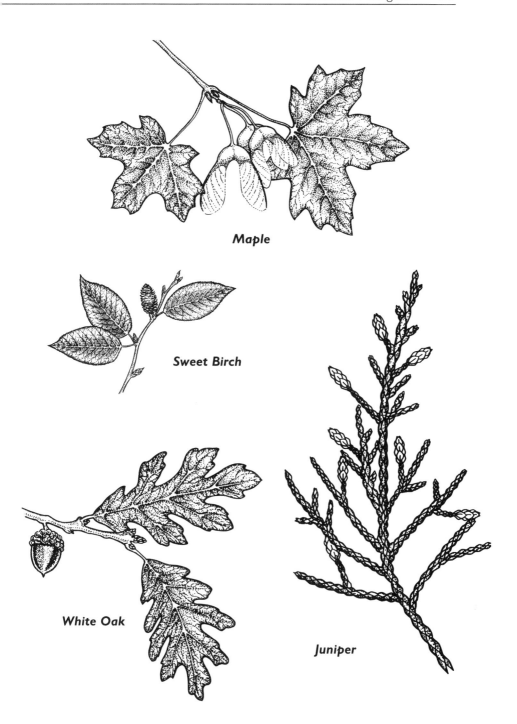

Maple

Sweet Birch

White Oak

Juniper

WHERE DO YOU LIVE?

The following descriptions of the pollen season reflect the longest probable time span in each region of the U.S. In actuality, the pollen season in any given region is likely to be shorter than indicated.

- **Northeastern, Southeastern and Central states.** Depending on the specific area, tree pollen — from birch, maple, ash and oak — may be common from February through June. Various grass pollens are predominant from May through August. Ragweed pollen is present from June through November.

- **Great Lakes region and Mountain states.** Trees such as oak and maple pollinate from March through June. Grasses produce pollen April through July. Ragweed pollen may be present from June through October.

- **Western states.** Although outdoor seasonal allergies certainly exist in the West, they may be less of a concern because of lower levels of pollen (particularly from ragweed) compared to other regions, as well as the higher altitudes of some areas. However, the intensity of tree and grass pollens in some parts of the West (California, the Southwest) can parallel those in the central U.S.

The charts on pages 30-33 provide a more detailed picture of the pollens that are most prevalent in your part of the country during certain times of the year.

Outdoor Molds

Many different types of molds lurk outdoors and may trigger many of the same seasonal symptoms that are typically associated with pollen. These outdoor molds are most likely to produce allergy-related problems from summer through autumn (July to November). They can cause symptoms as early as the spring thaw and as late as the last days of autumn. These microscopic fungi create allergy problems from their hiding places on fallen leaves and freshly-cut grass, and in damp, shady areas. They also can thrive in any decaying organic material, such as soil, and on trees, weeds, hay, straw and rotting wood. When the spores (seeds) from these molds become airborne, they may be breathed into the nose or land on the eyes. Mold spores or mold proteins can also be inhaled into the lungs and trigger asthma episodes.

If you have mold allergies, you may start to sniffle and wipe away tears whenever these spores are stirred up—for example, when you mow the lawn, rake leaves or even walk across a newly-cut lawn or through a pile of leaves. Symptoms can also appear when you go on a hayride, walk through a damp barn or go camping in the woods.

As with pollen, the levels of mold spores in the air (as well as indoors) will vary with the time of year and the weather conditions. At certain times in some areas, airborne mold levels will actually exceed the amount of pollen in the air. Molds can survive in extremely cold temperatures, and sometimes continue to flourish even after the first snow cover (although airborne spore levels tend to decline at that time). In the South and West, molds can be a year-round problem. While molds are found in all parts of the country, they occur in the highest concentrations in the grain-growing areas of the Midwest, attaching themselves to barley, corn and oats.

Although some molds become more problematic in windy and dry environments, others thrive when the air is damp. In general, however, the levels of mold spores in the air tend to be lower on cold

REGIONAL ALLERGENS

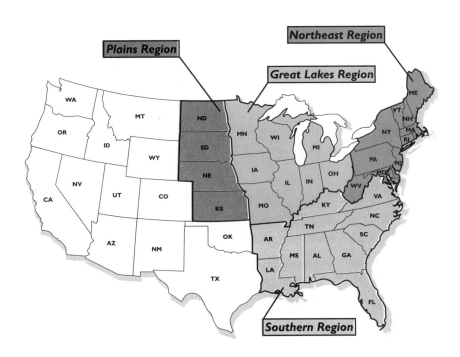

Predominant Pollen/Seasons

Northeast Region

Pollens	Jan	Feb	Mar	Apr	May	Jun	Jul	Aug	Sep	Oct	Nov	Dec
TREES												
Oak			‖‖‖‖‖‖‖‖‖‖‖‖‖‖‖‖‖‖‖‖‖‖‖‖‖‖									
Pine			‖‖‖‖‖‖‖‖‖‖‖‖‖‖‖‖‖‖‖‖‖‖‖‖‖‖									
Birch			‖‖‖‖‖‖‖‖‖‖‖‖‖‖‖‖‖‖‖‖‖‖‖‖‖‖									
GRASSES				‖‖‖‖‖‖‖‖‖‖‖‖‖‖‖‖‖‖‖‖‖‖‖‖								
WEEDS												
Ragweed							‖‖‖‖‖‖‖‖‖‖‖‖‖‖‖‖‖‖				
Plantain							‖‖‖‖‖‖‖‖‖‖‖‖‖‖‖‖‖‖				
Nettle							‖‖‖‖‖‖‖‖‖‖‖‖‖‖‖‖‖‖				

* Note: Trees, grasses and weeds do not pollinate at the same time or in the same sequence each year

Great Lakes Region

Pollens	Jan	Feb	Mar	Apr	May	Jun	Jul	Aug	Sep	Oct	Nov	Dec
TREES												
Elm			▓	▓	▓	▓						
Oak			▓	▓	▓	▓						
Maple			▓	▓	▓	▓						
GRASSES					▓	▓	▓					
WEEDS												
Ragweed							▓	▓	▓	▓		
Plantain							▓	▓	▓	▓		
Nettle							▓	▓	▓	▓		

Southern Region

Pollens	Jan	Feb	Mar	Apr	May	Jun	Jul	Aug	Sep	Oct	Nov	Dec
TREES												
Pecan		▓	▓	▓	▓							
Oak		▓	▓	▓	▓							
Cedar		▓	▓	▓	▓							
GRASSES	▓	▓	▓	▓	▓	▓	▓	▓	▓	▓	▓	▓
WEEDS												
Ragweed						▓	▓	▓	▓	▓	▓	
Plantain						▓	▓	▓	▓	▓	▓	
Nettle						▓	▓	▓	▓	▓	▓	

Plains Region

Pollens	Jan	Feb	Mar	Apr	May	Jun	Jul	Aug	Sep	Oct	Nov	Dec
TREES												
Oak			▓	▓	▓							
Cedar			▓	▓	▓							
Rye			▓	▓	▓							
GRASSES					▓	▓	▓					
WEEDS												
Ragweed							▓	▓	▓	▓		
Plantain							▓	▓	▓	▓		
Nettle							▓	▓	▓	▓		

Source: Surveillance Data Inc., 1998

REGIONAL ALLERGENS

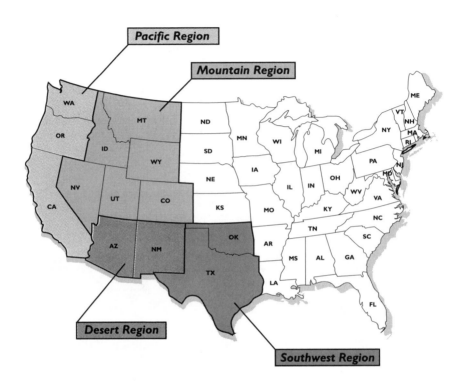

Predominant Pollen/Seasons

Pacific Region

Pollens	Jan	Feb	Mar	Apr	May	Jun	Jul	Aug	Sep	Oct	Nov	Dec
TREES												
Cedar		‖‖‖‖‖‖‖‖‖‖‖‖‖‖‖‖‖‖‖‖‖‖‖‖									
Walnut		‖‖‖‖‖‖‖‖‖‖‖‖‖‖‖‖‖‖‖‖‖‖‖‖									
Rye		‖‖‖‖‖‖‖‖‖‖‖‖‖‖‖‖‖‖‖‖‖‖‖‖									
GRASSES			‖‖								
WEEDS												
Ragweed				‖‖‖‖‖‖‖‖‖‖‖‖‖‖‖‖‖‖‖‖‖‖‖‖‖‖‖‖‖‖‖‖‖‖‖‖						
Chenopod				‖‖‖‖‖‖‖‖‖‖‖‖‖‖‖‖‖‖‖‖‖‖‖‖‖‖‖‖‖‖‖‖‖‖‖‖						
Sage				‖‖‖‖‖‖‖‖‖‖‖‖‖‖‖‖‖‖‖‖‖‖‖‖‖‖‖‖‖‖‖‖‖‖‖‖						

* Note: Trees, grasses and weeds do not pollinate at the same time or in the same sequence each year.

Mountain Region

Pollens	Jan	Feb	Mar	Apr	May	Jun	Jul	Aug	Sep	Oct	Nov	Dec
TREES												
Cedar			▓	▓								
Maple			▓	▓								
Oak			▓	▓								
GRASSES				▓	▓	▓						
WEEDS												
Ragweed							▓	▓	▓	▓	▓	
Tumbleweed							▓	▓	▓	▓	▓	
Chenopod							▓	▓	▓	▓	▓	

Desert Region

Pollens	Jan	Feb	Mar	Apr	May	Jun	Jul	Aug	Sep	Oct	Nov	Dec
TREES												
Cedar		▓	▓	▓								
Ash		▓	▓	▓								
Oak		▓	▓	▓								
GRASSES				▓	▓	▓	▓	▓	▓	▓		
WEEDS												
Ragweed			▓	▓	▓	▓	▓	▓	▓	▓	▓	▓
Chenopod			▓	▓	▓	▓	▓	▓	▓	▓	▓	▓
Sage			▓	▓	▓	▓	▓	▓	▓	▓	▓	▓

Southwest Region

Pollens	Jan	Feb	Mar	Apr	May	Jun	Jul	Aug	Sep	Oct	Nov	Dec
TREES												
Cedar	▓	▓	▓	▓	▓	▓						
Elm	▓	▓	▓	▓	▓	▓						
Oak	▓	▓	▓	▓	▓	▓						
GRASSES				▓	▓	▓	▓	▓	▓			
WEEDS												
Ragweed						▓	▓	▓	▓	▓		
Chenopod						▓	▓	▓	▓	▓		
Dock						▓	▓	▓	▓	▓		

Source: Surveillance Data Inc., 1998

rainy days, and at high altitudes; they are likely to be highest in humid conditions and *after* a rainstorm. Molds are particularly abundant in the fall and are responsible for the decaying of leaves and rotting of vegetative matter.

The risk of exposure to molds is highest near fields where crops (especially grains) are being grown, and in overgrown fields and pastures. Farm workers have a very high risk at times when threshing, baling and combining are taking place, because these activities release huge numbers of spores into the air.

For city-dwellers, gardening is a potential source of trouble, stirring large numbers of spores into the air when cutting grass, clearing brush and spreading mulch. For example, fusarium is a mold that thrives on wood chips commonly used in gardening.

Avoiding Problems with Outdoor Allergens

Even if you're prone to outdoor allergies, and you have no choice but to spend time outdoors, it is possible to eliminate or decrease your symptoms. In many cases this can be accomplished with only some relatively simple life-style changes. When those are not sufficient, your doctor can recommend medications to prevent or control the allergic reactions.

The first step is to identify the allergens that trigger your reactions and avoid them. Take that step, and your symptoms will probably decrease in severity, if not clear completely.

The following questionnaire will help you and your doctor to identify some specific outdoor allergy triggers or troublesome locations. Place a check mark by the statements that apply to you:

_____ My nose becomes congested or itchy, and I start to sneeze or develop a scratchy throat or wheeze when I rake leaves or clear brush. [mold]

_____ My symptoms flare whenever I mow the lawn. [pollen, mold]

_____ My symptoms are aggravated by simply walking in my front yard or backyard. [pollen]

_____ There are pollen-bearing trees or plants in my yard or neighborhood. [pollen]

_____ When I walk through a nearby park or go on a camping trip, my symptoms worsen. [pollen, mold]

_____ My symptoms occur when nearby crops are being harvested. [mold]

The following guidelines will help you avoid airborne pollen and mold spores:

• **Limit your time outdoors when pollen counts are high.** In general, you need to stay indoors during late morning and afternoon when pollen is most prevalent. Most ragweed pollen is dispersed into the air between 9 a.m. and 11 a.m.; however, certain grasses and weeds pollinate later in the afternoon. Also, stay indoors when the wind is blowing and the humidity is high.

- **Avoid areas outdoors where molds could accumulate.** Stay away from piles of leaves and soil. Also, clean up areas around your home where drainage problems cause pools or puddles of water to accumulate. Damp areas like these can encourage the growth of mold. Clean out the rain gutters, too; if leaves accumulate in them, they can become sites for mold growth.

- **Keep the windows in your home shut to prevent pollen and mold spores from drifting in.** Whether at home or in your car, keep the doors and windows closed when allergen levels are high. In the car, run the air conditioner on "recirculate." When outdoors, wear wraparound sunglasses to minimize pollen contact with your eyes. Air conditioning allows windows and doors to remain closed, thereby preventing pollens and mold spores from gaining entrance. If possible, use an air conditioning system continuously during the pollen season. Although many people open the windows of their homes at night, this may allow mold spores into the bedroom from the outdoors.

- **If you have been outdoors, shower (and wash your hair) before going to sleep.** Pollen gets trapped in your hair and on your skin when you are outdoors. Bathing and showering before you go to bed will wash the pollen away so it doesn't end up on your pillow and bedding, where it then can be easily inhaled.

- **Avoid hanging clothes and sheets out to dry during pollen season.** Pollen tends to "stick" to laundry on outdoor clotheslines. When you later wear clothes or use bedding dried this way, you are then exposed to that pollen. You can avoid this by using a hot-air clothes dryer or by drying your laundry indoors.

- **Have a nonallergic family member (or a gardener) mow the lawn and rake the leaves.** Cutting grass, raking and weeding stir up molds and pollens, propelling them into the air. If you can, pass on these chores to someone else who is not allergic. If you insist on doing yard work yourself, wear a particle mask that filters allergens. This kind of mask can be purchased at hardware stores or garden centers. When you come indoors afterward, leave your outer garments at the door to avoid tracking allergens throughout the house. Don't wear the same clothes again until they have been washed and the pollens removed. Shower immediately to get pollens and molds off your skin and out of your hair.

- **Exercise where and when pollens are least likely to affect you.** Don't exercise in parks where pollen-bearing trees and grass are prevalent. The best days for exercise are those that are overcast and free of winds. On high-pollen days, exercise indoors, at home or at a local fitness facility.

DON'T FEAR ALL THE FLOWERS

Not all trees, grasses and weeds pose problems for people with allergies. There are upwards of 700 species of trees in North America, but only about 10% of these have been associated with allergic rhinitis. Ironically, some of the most feared plants—the brightly flowering varieties—are the least likely to trigger allergic symptoms. The colorful flowers attract insects, and the pollen of roses and many other fragrant, colorful flowers tends to be heavy, waxy and sticky. It is therefore less likely to become airborne, compared to the finer, lighter pollens released by trees, weeds and grasses. As a result, allergies to these brightly flowering plants are relatively rare, except among florists and gardeners, who are exposed to them constantly.

- **Keep indoor/outdoor pets (for example, dogs, cats) out of your bedroom during pollen/mold seasons.** Pets can carry allergens from outdoors on their coats. In your bedroom, these pollens or molds can become airborne, or they can be directly transferred to beds, chairs, carpets and everything else the pets come into contact with. These allergens can linger—and cause symptoms—long after the pets have left the room.

- **Schedule your vacations during your city's peak allergy season, and try to spend them in places that are less likely to trigger allergy symptoms.** If you can get out of town when allergen levels are high, you'll be more comfortable. Some people have taken this strategy to the next stage: When allergy symptoms become intolerable, they pack their belongings and move to another part of the country. But this is costly, inconvenient—and often ineffective. While you may be escaping the pollens that cause sneezing and sniffling at your first home, there's no guarantee that you won't encounter new allergens that cause problems at the next location. It could take several years of seasonal exposure to the new allergens before your body develops IgE antibodies against them.

IS RAGWEED
IN YOUR COMMUNITY?

Ragweed is the dominant airborne allergen east of the Mississippi. It is particularly intense in the Northern and Central U.S. The East Coast is in a moderate ragweed belt. Concentrations in the South are lighter. The Rocky Mountains tend to limit the spread of ragweed westward. However, it is found in parts of the West, like the Salt Lake area.

Working with Your Doctor

If you are not able to eliminate your symptoms or reduce them to a tolerable level with the actions described in this chapter, it's important to discuss the use of medications with your doctor. Some medications can be used preventively to block the allergic reaction before it gets started. Other medications are used therapeutically to reverse the changes that occur during an allergic reaction.

You will find a complete discussion of allergy medications in Chapter 5. This information will prepare you for a discussion with your doctor about which medication is most appropriate in your particular case. Do not be discouraged if you have tried allergy medications in the past and not been pleased with the outcome. Prescription antihistamines are available that can relieve allergy symptoms without the drowsiness that may be associated with older antihistamines (such as over-the-counter antihistamines).

The following questionnaires will help your doctor review the preventive steps you have already taken. This will help the doctor develop a plan for further action that can include additional life-style measures and medications, if appropriate.

SYMPTOM RESPONSE CHART

Before I took steps to minimize my reaction to outdoor allergens, my symptoms were:

Symptom	Severity* (before changes)
runny nose	_____
sneezing	_____
itchy nose	_____
postnasal drip	_____
nasal congestion	_____
cough	_____
itchy, watery eyes	_____
headaches	_____
fatigue	_____
other (_____)	_____

I have taken the following steps to avoid outdoor allergens:

_____

_____

_____

_____

_____

_____

_____

SYMPTOM RESPONSE CHART

After implementing strategies for preventing contact with outdoor allergens, my symptoms have changed in the following way:

Symptom	Severity* (after changes)
runny nose	_____
sneezing	_____
itchy nose	_____
postnasal drip	_____
nasal congestion	_____
cough	_____
itchy, watery eyes	_____
headaches	_____
fatigue	_____
other (_____)	_____

*Severity Scale (0-3 Scale):

0 = none

1 = mild

2 = moderate

3 = severe

Chapter 3

Allergies in Your Home

If you think of your home as a haven from allergens, think again. From the kitchen to the bedroom, and the attic to the basement, potential allergens are probably just a sneeze away.

Unlike many outdoor allergens, which tend to be present seasonally (especially in the spring and fall), indoor allergens are more likely to be present year-round, and thus are likely to generate allergic symptoms throughout the year. Hence, allergies triggered by these predominantly "indoor" allergens are often referred to as "perennial" allergies.

Since most of us spend 90% of our life indoors, our exposure to indoor allergens — over time — can be great. That's why some people with perennial allergies may have such severe symptoms. It's also why you must be so meticulous when implementing an avoidance program aimed at indoor allergens. For example, when you consider that your head lies on the pillow for eight hours each night, you can't afford to have any allergens lurking on or in that pillow. If you're conscientious and follow the self-management guidelines described later in this chapter, you can significantly reduce, or perhaps even eliminate, your exposure to these allergens and your risk of an out-right allergic attack.

The primary indoor allergens that cause symptoms are:
- Dust mites and the particles they leave behind
- Molds
- Pet dander, saliva and urine
- Cockroaches and the particles they leave behind

Dust Mites

If you're a finicky housekeeper without an allergy, house dust is just an eyesore. But if you're also allergy-prone, house dust can actually cause itchy, red, sore eyes—as well as a runny nose, sneezing and wheezing.

Typical house dust contains all kinds of materials in addition to the soil carried in on the soles of your shoes. It may also include many allergens, including remnants of plant matter as well as dust mites—tiny, eight-legged creatures which can be seen only under a microscope.

Dust mites are the real culprits in dust-related allergies. It's not the "dirt" in dust that causes the trouble, but the mites—or more specifically, the proteins in their fecal matter and their decaying or decomposing body parts—which are responsible for a large share of the allergic reactions from which people suffer.

The mites hide out in places like carpeting, furniture cushions, mattresses and pillows—wherever dust and human skin cells collect. When something stirs the mites and their even tinier droppings into the air that you breathe, it can trigger a stuffy nose and sneezing—or even worse. (That's exactly what happens when you put your head down on your pillow or sit down on a sofa.)

Dust mites thrive especially well in humid and warm conditions (70 to 80 degrees Fahrenheit), even during the cold of winter when the heater is humming. They are much less common in dry climates or at high altitudes. (Mile-high Denver has far fewer dust mites than humid St. Louis or Chicago.)

Mites could not thrive were it not for their human "hosts." They feed on dead skin cells shed by people. For that reason, the mites tend to be particularly prevalent in carpeting, mattresses and bed pillows, and in sofa cushions and upholstered chairs, because that's where humans spend many hours a day (shedding dead skin cells all the time). The mites thrive in these locations because they have a constantly replenished source of food. Mites are scarce on venetian blinds or other smooth surfaces (even if they are "dusty"), because they have no food source there.

Just "cleaning house" won't necessarily free you of a dust mite problem because the mites hide or hang on with their claws where you can't see them: inside pillows, mattresses and sofa cushions; within the weave of blankets; and down low in the pile of carpets. Just sitting on the couch, or walking on the carpet, or putting your head on the pillow stirs the dust mite allergens (including their powdery fecal matter) into the air you breathe. That's why some people complain of a stuffy nose, watery eyes and sneezing every morning after rolling around on the pillow all night, or every evening after hours of relaxing in their favorite overstuffed chair.

When You're Allergic to Dust Mites...

As problematic as dust mites can be, removing them from your household is much more challenging than merely bringing out the feather duster (which only stirs the allergenic particles up into the air, where they can cause trouble for you) and the vacuum cleaner (which can become a problem, also, if you don't use good equipment and if the bag isn't changed frequently). You also may have to change the way you furnish your home. If you're conscientious, however, you can make headway against these microscopic critters. It is usually easiest and most effective to focus first on the allergic person's bedroom. Once that room is "allergen-proofed," focus on the family or living room, where the most time is spent.

Here are some proven strategies to decrease dust mite allergen levels in your home:

- Cover all mattresses and box springs with airtight plastic or vinyl allergen-proof encasings. They trap the mites inside, and keep them from triggering symptoms. They also cut off the supply of food (dead human skin cells that have been shed) for the mites. For extra protection, place fabric-reinforced tape over the zipper. Clean the outside of the casings regularly with a damp cloth.

- Wash all bed pillows weekly in hot water or cover with allergen-proof encasings.

- Use polyester-fiber-filled pillows and comforters.

- Do not use feather or down pillows and down-filled blankets or comforters.

- Store clean clothing and bedding in a dry environment.

- Wash all bedding weekly—including sheets, pillowcases, blankets and comforters—in hot (not warm) water. At temperatures of 130 degrees Fahrenheit or more, dust mite allergen levels can be lowered by over 90%; washing in colder temperatures allows them to survive. Hot-air drying alone is not enough.

DO YOU NEED AN AIR FILTER?

Your home's heating, cooling and ventilation systems can circulate allergens throughout the house. For that reason, you may wish to consider using air filters to cut down the movement of airborne allergens throughout your home. HEPA and electrostatic filters trap not only dust, but also pollen, mold spores and pet dander (ordinary furnace filters are not effective for this). It is important to remember that air filters remove only airborne particles but will not remove dust/allergens that have settled on surfaces or are present in bedding, carpets or furniture. Therefore, they are generally ineffective for house dust mite allergens, but may help with animal dander, mold and tobacco smoke. Thus, continuous use of filters in a forced-air system may decrease your exposure to animal dander, mold and tobacco smoke, thereby decreasing certain allergy symptoms.

One particularly efficient type of air cleaner, called a HEPA (High Efficiency Particulate Air) filter, consists of a complex network of fine glass fibers that collect allergen particles. When a HEPA filter is incorporated into the heating and air conditioning ducts, it can generally reduce the levels of certain allergens in your home.

Another filter commonly in use is the electrostatic filter, which gives airborne particles a negative charge as they enter the unit. This causes the

• Remove wall-to-wall carpeting from areas where the allergic person in your family spends time, such as the bedroom. (Carpets, particularly shag carpets, are an ideal site for dust mites to congregate.) Hardwood, tile or linoleum floors are a better choice, with *washable* throw rugs, if desired.

---

particles to cling to positively-charged plates. Electrostatic filters are not as efficient as HEPA filters in trapping smaller particles. Electrostatic filters also must be rinsed frequently to continue to attract dust. Check your manufacturer's instructions for efficient use.

Freestanding air cleaners are available if your house doesn't have a central air and heating system. You should choose a HEPA unit that is capable of recirculating the air in the room several times each hour. Although desktop models are available, you may need a larger one to do a good job. If you use a desktop model, it should be placed on a table and not on the floor where it would disturb settled dust.

The Asthma & Allergy Foundation of America recommends that you ask the following questions when shopping for a portable air cleaner:

• What substances will the cleaner remove from the air? What substances will it not affect?
• Can the unit clean the air in your room every four to six minutes?
• How difficult is it to change and clean the air filters? (Ask for a demonstration.) How often do you have to change the filters? How much do replacement filters cost and are they easily available?
• How much noise does the unit make? Turn it on and try it. Is it quiet enough to run while you sleep?

- If you decide to keep your carpeting, have it vacuumed often. However, unless you wear a special mask (available at most hardware stores) to filter the air during vacuuming, have someone who is not allergic do it. Keep in mind that dust particles stay in the air as long as two hours after being disturbed (for example, by vacuuming), so you should try to stay out of any room that has been vacuumed for at least that long. Also, be aware that although steam-cleaning does reduce the levels of mite allergens, it does so for only about one month.

- When furnishing your home — particularly the bedrooms and other rooms where family members spend the most time — avoid items that are likely to accumulate dust mites. That means selecting vinyl, wooden, metal or leather chairs rather than upholstered ones.

- Choose washable toys made of rubber, plastic, metal or wood for your children.

- If your children have stuffed animals, keep these toys in the freezer in bags when not in use. Purchase stuffed animals only if they are washable in hot water, and wash them regularly.

- Keep your home well-ventilated. Weather permitting, open the windows for at least a few minutes several times a day. During pollen season, use window filters to help keep pollens out while the windows are open.

- Use central air conditioning or dehumidifiers to help control humidity levels. Indoor humidity should be kept below 50%. A relative humidity of 20 - 30% is most comfortable to the nose and skin, and yet does not encourage dust mite growth. (At higher levels, dust mites are more likely to thrive.)

- If you use dehumidifiers, remember to clean them often to prevent mold growth.

- Do not use room fans, which only stir up dust.

- Avoid living in the basement.

WHERE DO INDOOR MOLDS LURK?

Molds are really tiny plants, so it's not surprising that they thrive in damp places. The following indoor sites are common places where molds are found. All of them offer dark or humid environments where molds can grow:

- Bathrooms, showers
- Humidifiers, vaporizers, air conditioners

- Refrigerators (including drip pans)
- Mattresses

- Chair and sofa cushions
- Soil of houseplants

- Under carpets
- Under and behind washing machines

- Water-damaged wallpaper
- Garbage pails

- Plumbing fixtures
- Foam pillows

- Window and door frames, ledges
- Fireplace logs

- Basements
- Crawl spaces and attics

Molds

Just the mention of the word "mold" makes some people cringe, as they recall images of green growths on stale bread, old fruit or spoiled food. For others, the picture is one of fuzzy mold clusters in the dark corners of a basement. In fact, there are thousands of different molds, and many are actually "human-friendly" — for example, the molds that produce disease-fighting antibiotics, such as penicillin.

Molds are really just very tiny plants. Like dust mites, mold spores cannot be seen by the naked eye. They only become visible when conditions are right for their growth and multiplication, producing "colonies" that are large enough to see (at that point, you may also be able to detect their musty odor). Also, like dust mites, molds survive by feeding on organic material in the environment, such as plant particles or animal matter.

Molds thrive in dark, humid environments. Dampness, in fact, is mold's greatest ally. That's why it is so commonly found in basements, crawl spaces, bathrooms and kitchens, especially in refrigerators. Other sites where mold commonly grows include garbage bins, indoor plant soil, sofa cushions, mattresses, window and door frames, humidifiers and under carpets that have been laid on concrete floors.

Molds create allergy problems by dispersing tiny spores (reproductive cells) into the air. This can be triggered by the slightest breeze or draft, as occurs when you close a refrigerator door or sweep behind a washing machine. If these spores land on organic matter that provides a source of nutrition, they begin to multiply. And if you're allergic and mold spores land inside your nose when you inhale, they can trigger an allergic reaction.

People in certain occupations are more likely to encounter mold spores as part of their jobs. These include florists and greenhouse employees (it's not the flowers, but the constant humidity or moisture at the worksite that causes the problem), bakers, butchers and wallpaper hangers. For people who are allergy-prone, these jobs can become a chronic source of symptoms.

When You're Allergic to Molds...

Finding and eradicating molds from your home isn't nearly as difficult as getting dust under control, although it still will take some conscientious effort. The key is to identify and eliminate dampness throughout your house. Here's how to do it:

- Inspect dark, inadequately ventilated areas of the house, which are the places where humidity is most likely to be high and indoor molds are most likely to thrive. Look at the bathrooms, kitchen (including refrigerator water pans), laundry room, attic and crawl spaces for leaks, dampness, mildew and molds. Also check the windowsills and panes, garbage pails, houseplant soil, wallpaper, carpets, rugs, firewood and old books.

- Use air conditioning and dehumidifiers to decrease dampness and humidity, especially in basements.

- If you don't have an air conditioner and live in a relatively dry climate, keep windows open to maintain circulation.

- Clean dehumidifiers and air conditioners often so they don't become breeding grounds themselves for mold.

- Clean and then dry potentially troublesome areas of your kitchen and bathroom, such as shower stalls and curtains, bath mats, soap dishes, tubs, tiles, toilets, kitchen and bathroom sinks, plumbing fixtures, floors and walls.

- Keep your bathroom, kitchen and laundry room well-ventilated at all times.

- Dry off the shower walls and bathroom floor after bathing.

- Clean all mold-containing surfaces with chlorine bleach, disinfectants or commercial fungicides, which can destroy mold and mildew. An effective bleach mixture consists of 1 part bleach and 10 parts water. Before using these cleaners or bleach, check the color-fastness of the surface.

- Empty and clean garbage pails frequently. Don't allow moisture to collect in them.

- Throw out stale food.

- Ventilate closets.

- Dry out damp shoes before placing them in the closet.

- Remove old wallpaper, particularly if it shows signs of mildew, and re-paper using mold-resistant glue, or apply paint instead.

- In rooms that tend to become damp, choose a paint with additives that block mold formation.

- If your home is prone to mold formation, dry-clean rather than steam-clean the carpets.

- Remove any carpeting in the bathrooms and carpeting on cement slab flooring.

- Get rid of aquariums.

- Minimize potted plants in your home (watering the plants disperses mold spores into the air) and keep them out of the bedrooms completely.

- Never place damp clothes in a laundry hamper.

Cockroaches

Can anything send shivers down your spine more quickly than the sight of a cockroach racing across the kitchen or bedroom floor? Though unpleasant to see, it is not those intact living creatures that cause problems for people with allergies. The allergic symptoms are triggered by the eggs and excrement these creatures leave in their wake, and by the powdery residue of their carcasses after they die. These tiny elements—when inhaled—appear to be a common cause of allergic respiratory symptoms, skin rashes and asthma episodes.

Roaches are especially common in city apartment complexes and wherever living conditions are crowded. Their favorite—though by no means exclusive—home within your home is in the kitchen, especially on the floor and in the cupboards. One recent study found that cockroach allergen was 50 times more common in kitchens than in bedrooms and upholstered furniture. Even in homes where cockroaches hadn't been reported as a problem by residents, researchers detected evidence of cockroach allergen in some of the kitchens, bedrooms and living rooms they tested.

To put your mind at ease, however, cockroaches are not a sign of an unkempt home. Americans spend more money trying to eradicate cockroaches than any other household pest, and still they are nearly everywhere. Roaches find a way to thrive in even the tidiest houses, eating virtually anything to survive, including food scraps, paper — even each other! They hide out in dark, warm places, and run for cover when they find themselves in the light. For at least 10 million Americans, they are highly allergenic. A study at Kaiser Permanente in San Francisco tested 180 patients prone to allergies, and found that 40% had allergic reactions to cockroach allergens.

When You're Allergic to Cockroaches...

You not only need to kill existing roaches, but also eliminate the residue of those that have already died. Think about the places where cockroaches flourish; those should be the areas in which you wage your household war against roaches. Here are some ways to help you gain the upper hand:

- Keep your kitchen clean and free of leftover food or food particles on the counters and floor. Keep all food covered, preferably in airtight cans and containers.

- Wash and dry dirty dishes immediately after meals.

- Empty garbage daily.

- Take newspapers outside before they accumulate. Don't collect paper grocery bags or cardboard boxes in the house, either.

- Use large roach traps containing a chemical called *hydramethylnon* or insecticides like boric acid powder in the kitchen or other parts of the house where you've found roaches. (Boric acid is typically placed in kitchen cupboards, under the stove and refrigerator, and other places where roaches turn up.) Check manufacturers' instructions for frequency of replacement of traps. **Remember to read the labels carefully, as some of these products can be poisonous and cause a hazard to pets and small children.**

- Keep moisture and dampness under control. In some very humid apartments this can be accomplished by opening the windows. Repair leaky faucets and pipes. Wrap pipes with insulation if moisture condenses on the pipes.

- Call an exterminator if these efforts fail. Individuals with asthma should not be present during insect spraying and for at least two hours after as chemicals (such as pyrethrins) can trigger an asthma episode. You may want to find out which chemicals the exterminator will be using, then check with your doctor about the safety of those chemicals.

Pets and Other Animals

For many individuals, life without a dog or a cat is unthinkable. Unfortunately, many of these same people are allergic to their household animals. Your irreplaceable pooch may excel at fetching the morning paper, but he might also be responsible for making your nose drip or your eyes itch. In fact, some people can't be in the same room with a dog or a cat without developing allergic symptoms — in some cases, very severe symptoms.

Even so, about half of all homes in America have one or more cats or dogs — a surprising statistic considering that dog or cat allergies occur in up to 10% of the population. If you have asthma, your chances of having a pet allergy are even higher, with the risk increasing to 20-30%. Allergies to cats are twice as common as those to dogs.

Contrary to common belief, it's not the pet's hair that causes the allergic reaction. The hair itself acts only as a carrier for allergy-causing proteins. The problem is caused by an immune reaction to proteins found in the millions of flaky skin scales (dander) shed by the animal each day. The pet's saliva (salivary protein) and urine (urinary protein) may also be significant sources of allergens. All of these allergens can be inhaled into human lungs, or settle in the nose or the eyes.

In the case of cats, the primary allergen is secreted by glands in their skin. It is also present in their saliva. In a typical scenario, a cat will have the allergen clinging to its fur; then this allergen will float through the air when the animal moves or when it is brushed, petted or bathed. These allergens are microscopic and may be airborne continuously in a home with a cat, so they can cause severe allergic symptoms, even without any physical contact with the cat itself. Highly allergic people can even experience symptoms when entering a home where a cat used to live but no longer does; that's because allergens can linger for many months — even years. This is especially common in apartments or homes that have carpets and upholstered furniture, which serve as hiding places for pet allergens.

Some research suggests that dogs are generally less allergenic than cats, although some people are still highly allergic to man's best friend. The allergenic proteins in dogs also come from saliva and skin. Some people say that they're allergic to certain breeds of dogs, but not others. In fact, all dogs are capable of causing allergy-related problems, so if you're allergic to dogs, don't expect a short-haired breed to pose fewer problems than a long-haired one.

Keep in mind that the offending animal may be something other than a dog or a cat. If you or your children have a guinea pig, gerbil, mouse, hamster or rabbit, for example, its urinary protein in particular can trigger allergic symptoms. Farm and barnyard animals, such as horses and cows, can cause allergies, too. Even pet birds, particularly droppings on their feathers, can produce symptoms. In fact, most (but not all) pets can trigger an allergic response in people who are sensitized.

When You're Allergic to Pets...

If you're allergic to a household pet, the best advice is try to find a new home for it. Anything less, and you cannot count on freedom from allergic symptoms.

Some allergy-prone people believe that keeping the pet outdoors will solve the problem. This may help to some degree, but will not eliminate your exposure to pet allergens completely. Studies show that families with an outdoor dog or cat have higher levels of animal allergens in their homes than do pet-free households, even if the animal never comes inside (family members may carry the pet allergens into the house on their clothes). Restricting pets to just one or two rooms in the home isn't the solution, either, since their allergens can spread throughout the house on clothing or via heating

PREVENTING ALLERGIES IN CHILDREN

Whether the allergic person in your family is an adult or a child, the environmental-control strategies described in this chapter should help to minimize allergy symptoms. Some allergists also advise taking another step:

When a baby is born into a family that already has a strong history of allergies, even if the infant hasn't manifested any signs of allergies yet, you can assume that his or her chances of developing allergies are high. Rather than waiting for allergic symptoms to appear, and then making appropriate changes in your home, you can take some commonsense preventive steps.

Remember, children aren't born with allergies; they're born with the *potential* to develop them. Factors like exposure to allergens will play a key role in whether they do, in fact, become allergic. So if your family has a strong history of allergies, you can reduce a child's exposure to potential allergens by removing bedroom carpeting and replacing it with linoleum or a hardwood floor with a washable area rug. Use dust mite-proof covers on the child's bed, and avoid feather pillows and comforters. Also, don't get the family a dog or a cat; if there's never a pet in the house, your youngster will have a decreased probability of having a pet allergy.

ducts (although barring the pet from your bedroom is far better than doing nothing).

Even if you make the decision to put your pet up for adoption, the challenge isn't over yet. Remember, animal allergens can linger in households for months (sometimes for more than a year) in carpets, upholstered furniture and mattresses. Repeated vacuuming may help, although it won't reach into the lower levels of the carpets. Steam-cleaning is a better option. However, don't expect to have an allergen-free home overnight.

For some families, giving away their pet is an unacceptable option. If you fit this profile and insist on keeping your pet, there are ways to at least minimize exposure to animal allergens and make life more tolerable for allergy-prone family members. For example:

- Keep your pet outdoors most of the time. Your veterinarian can advise you regarding a shelter to protect the animal from the elements.

- When your dog or cat is indoors, keep it in a room (like the kitchen) that doesn't have carpeting or upholstered furniture. If the animal has access to other rooms, get rid of the carpets and upholstered furniture in those rooms, replacing the carpet with hardwood or linoleum floors.

- Make the bedrooms off limits for your pet, and keep the bedroom doors shut to ensure that a wandering pet doesn't sneak in. Even brief visits to your bedroom (or any room) by an animal will leave allergens there, long after the pet has left (cat allergen is also quite sticky, adhering to things like clothes and walls). Keep in mind that you probably spend more hours a day in your bedroom than in any other room in your house; children spend as much as one-half of their lives — sometimes more — in their bedrooms.

- Provide your dog or cat with its own bed; if it sleeps in yours, you are asking for trouble.

DOES YOUR CHILD'S SCHOOL TRIGGER ALLERGIES?

You can work hard to minimize the allergens that your child is exposed to at home, but you have much less control over his/her school setting. Still, if your child is experiencing allergic reactions at school, you should visit the school and classroom, look for potential problems, and ask the principal and teachers to cooperate by making the educational environment as allergen-free as possible.

As you review the list below, place a check mark beside those steps that may be appropriate at your child's school.

_____ Remove pets (for example, guinea pigs, gerbils, mice) from the classroom.

_____ Avoid keeping piles of newspapers—and the mold they attract—in the classroom.

_____ Check books and bookshelves frequently for mold growth and dust to prevent accumulation.

_____ Keep room closets free of dust-accumulating items, old clothes and moisture sources.

_____ Avoid conducting physical education or other activities in open areas or fields that may be sites of pollinating plants or molds.

_____ Remove plants from the classroom.

_____ Provide pillows with allergen-proof encasings for preschoolers who take naps at school; avoid feather pillows and down quilts.

_____ Provide for adequate fresh-air ventilation in the classroom.

Although some parents of nonallergic children may protest, stress the importance of making these changes.

- Install a good air cleaner in your home, such as a HEPA (High Efficiency Particulate Air) filter unit, which can significantly reduce levels of airborne pet allergens. (Remember, a significant portion of cat allergen will stay suspended in the air up to 18 to 24 hours once disturbed.)

- If you have a hamster, mouse or other rodent pet, recruit an allergy-free person to clean the cage.

- Wash your pet about once a week, which will get rid of at least some of the allergens that linger in its fur. Tepid water is fine; soap isn't necessary. Although cats sometimes protest attempts to wash them, those that have been bathed since they were kittens tend to be much more cooperative. Even an older cat can become used to bathing after a few sessions. The introduction of a cat to bathing should proceed slowly — from a few drops of water on its fur to a full rinse. Rewarding the cat with treats is helpful. Have a nonallergic family member wash and groom the cat. Several studies have found that regular washing gradually reduces the levels of airborne allergens shed by pets, but the reduction in the overall allergen level in the home has been very limited.

If you finally decide to find another home for your dog or cat, take steps to ease the emotional withdrawal you might feel. There actually are a few allergy-free animals you can live with. Although they may not fit your image of the ideal family pet, at least they'll keep you from sneezing and sniffling. These include turtles, lizards and hermit crabs. You may not be able to take them for a walk, but if you need to stay away from dogs, cats, rodents and birds, these animals can provide a safe alternative.

WHERE ELSE ARE YOU ALLERGIC?

Your home isn't the only indoor setting where allergens can cause problems. If you have allergies, you may develop symptoms in many of the places you go. Here are a few other common troublesome sites:

SITE	COMMON PROBLEMS
Theaters	dust mites, mold, pet allergens on seats (carried in on the clothes of others)
Veterinarian offices	pet allergens
Farms	dust mites, mold, pollen, animal dander
Nurseries	pollen, mold
Libraries, bookstores	dust mites, mold
Schools	dust mites, mold, pet allergens
Offices	dust mites, mold, pollen (from plants)
Antique stores	dust mites, mold

Indoor Pollen Exposures

Plant pollen is associated primarily with outdoor allergies. But, although pollen usually originates outdoors, it can also drift into your home through open windows and doors, or piggyback its way inside, clinging to your clothing or hiding in your hair.

For a "refresher course" on pollens, turn to page 19. In the meantime, to minimize pollen risks inside your home, keep all the windows closed throughout pollen season and — if available — use the air conditioner. Before you come indoors, take off your jacket or sweater and leave it by the door; then take a shower, wash your hair thoroughly (pollen clings to it), and put on clean clothes. These simple steps could save you from prolonged exposure to aggravating allergens after you come inside.

Indoor Irritants ("The Other Allergies")

Many people describe having "allergic" reactions after indoor exposure to substances such as tobacco smoke, perfumes, soaps, aerosols, cleaning fluids, detergents and pastes. As discomforting as these episodes may feel, they are not true *allergic* reactions; the symptoms are not being caused by IgE. Rather, they're your body's response to *irritants.* Of course, when your nose is running, your eyes are tearing, and you're rapidly depleting a complete box of tissue, it probably doesn't matter to you whether you're reacting to an allergen or an irritant.

Avoidance of these irritants is the only effective way to deal with this problem. Allergy medicines won't quiet the symptoms because the underlying reaction isn't allergic in nature.

Taking Action

To get rid of your allergy symptoms, you've got to eliminate repeated (and often prolonged) exposure to allergens. Here are the key steps for allergen-fighting in your home: 1) Prevent allergens from entering your home (for example, keep pets outdoors); 2) Create obstacles to those allergens over which you really have no direct control, but that can sneak into your home (for instance, take steps to keep plant pollen out of the house by closing your windows, particularly on windy days).

Go through your house, room-by-room, completing the following check list to identify potential problems.

Living Room\Family Room	Yes	No
• Are carpets vacuumed frequently and cleaned regularly?		
• Do you have concrete floors under carpeting?		
• Do you have upholstered furniture that can harbor dust mites?		
• Are there throw pillows that can collect dust?		
• Is there visible mold on window and door frames and ledges?		
• Do you have an air conditioning unit that may be harboring mold?		
• Are there leaks that contribute to dampness and mold growth?		
• Do you have houseplants in the room?		
• During pollen season, are windows left open, allowing pollen to enter the room?		
• Do pets spend time in the living room or family room?		
• Is there a fish aquarium in which mold can grow?		

Bedroom #1		
• Are carpets vacuumed frequently and cleaned regularly?		
• Do you have concrete floors under carpeting?		
• Do you have upholstered furniture that can harbor dust mites?		
• Is there visible mold on window and door frames and ledges?		

	Yes	No
• Do you have an air conditioning unit that may be harboring mold?		
• Are there leaks that contribute to dampness and mold growth?		
• Do you have houseplants in the room?		
• During pollen season, are windows left open, allowing pollen to enter the room?		
• Have mattresses, box springs and pillows been encased in allergen-proof covers?		
• Do you have feather pillows or down comforters on the beds?		
• Is clothing stored in a dry environment?		
• Are the doors of clothes closets kept shut to keep out dust?		
• Do pets spend time in the bedroom?		
• Are humidifiers or vaporizers used in the bedroom and is mold growing in or around them?		
• Are there stuffed animals, stuffed toys or throw pillows that invite dust mites?		

Bedroom #2

	Yes	No
• Are carpets vacuumed frequently and cleaned regularly?		
• Do you have concrete floors under carpeting?		
• Do you have upholstered furniture that can harbor dust mites?		
• Is there visible mold on window and door frames and ledges?		
• Do you have an air conditioning unit that may be harboring mold?		
• Are there leaks that contribute to dampness and mold growth?		
• Do you have houseplants in the room?		
• During pollen season, are windows left open, allowing pollen to enter the room?		

	Yes	No
• Have mattresses, box springs and pillows been encased in allergen-proof covers?		
• Do you have feather pillows or down comforters on the beds?		
• Is clothing stored in a dry environment?		
• Are the doors of clothes closets kept shut to keep out dust?		
• Do pets spend time in the bedroom?		
• Are humidifiers or vaporizers used in the bedroom and is mold growing in or around them?		
• Are there stuffed animals, stuffed toys or throw pillows that invite dust mites?		

Bedroom #3

	Yes	No
• Are carpets vacuumed frequently and cleaned regularly?		
• Do you have concrete floors under carpeting?		
• Do you have upholstered furniture that can harbor dust mites?		
• Is there visible mold on window and door frames and ledges?		
• Do you have an air conditioning unit that may be harboring mold?		
• Are there leaks that contribute to dampness and mold growth?		
• Do you have houseplants in the room?		
• During pollen season, are windows left open, allowing pollen to enter the room?		
• Have mattresses, box springs and pillows been encased in allergen-proof covers?		
• Do you have feather pillows or down comforters on the beds?		
• Is clothing stored in a dry environment?		
• Are the doors of clothes closets kept shut to keep out dust?		
• Do pets spend time in the bedroom?		

	Yes	No

• Are humidifiers or vaporizers used in the bedroom and is mold growing in or around them?

• Are there stuffed animals, stuffed toys or throw pillows that invite dust mites?

Kitchen

• Do you have upholstered furniture that can harbor dust mites?

• Is there visible mold on window and door frames and ledges?

• Do you have an air conditioning unit that may be harboring mold?

• Are there leaks in the plumbing or the roof that contribute to dampness and mold growth?

• Do you have houseplants in the room?

• During pollen season, are windows left open, allowing pollen to enter the room?

• Is food kept in airtight containers and cans?

• Have you overlooked throwing out moldy or stale food that is in the refrigerator or cupboards?

• Are there food scraps on floors or countertops that could possibly attract cockroaches?

• Are garbage containers emptied daily?

• Is mold growing on garbage receptacles?

• Is the drip pan of your self-defrosting refrigerator emptied and cleaned regularly?

• Are there signs of mold under the sink, or in or around the refrigerator or dishwasher?

• Do pets spend time in the kitchen?

• Have you seen any cockroaches?

• Is the stove fan regularly used and vented to the outdoors?

	Yes	No

Bathroom #1

• Are rugs vacuumed frequently and cleaned regularly?

• Do you have concrete floors under carpeting?

• Is there visible mold on window and door frames and ledges?

• Do you have an air conditioning unit that may be harboring mold?

• Are there leaks in the plumbing or the roof that contribute to dampness and mold growth?

• Do you have houseplants in the room?

• During pollen season, are windows left open, allowing pollen to enter the room?

• Is there mold in or around the shower?

• Is there mold in or around the tub?

• Is there mold on soap dishes?

• Is there mold under the sink?

• Is there mold around the toilet?

• Is there mold on the floors, walls, wallpaper or ceiling?

• Are bath mats picked up and dried after each bath or shower?

• Are damp clothes or towels placed in the hamper?

• Is the bathroom well-ventilated?

• Does the bathroom have carpeting that could attract mold?

Bathroom #2

• Are rugs vacuumed frequently and cleaned regularly?

• Do you have concrete floors under carpeting?

• Is there visible mold on window and door frames and ledges?

	Yes	No
• Do you have an air conditioning unit that may be harboring mold?		
• Are there leaks in the plumbing or the roof that contribute to dampness and mold growth?		
• Do you have houseplants in the room?		
• During pollen season, are windows left open, allowing pollen to enter the room?		
• Is there mold in or around the shower?		
• Is there mold in or around the tub?		
• Is there mold on soap dishes?		
• Is there mold under the sink?		
• Is there mold around the toilet?		
• Is there mold on the floors, walls, wallpaper or ceiling?		
• Are bath mats picked up and dried after each bath or shower?		
• Are damp clothes or towels placed in the hamper?		
• Is the bathroom well-ventilated?		
• Does the bathroom have carpeting that could attract mold?		

Basement

	Yes	No
• Are carpets vacuumed frequently and cleaned regularly?		
• Do you have concrete floors under carpeting?		
• Do you have upholstered furniture that can harbor dust mites?		
• Is there visible mold on window and door frames and ledges?		
• Do you have an air conditioning unit that may be harboring mold?		
• Are there leaks in the home that contribute to dampness and mold growth?		

	Yes	No

• Do you have houseplants in the basement?

• During pollen season, are windows left open, allowing pollen
  to enter the basement?

• Are there damp areas that are harboring mold?

• Does flooding occur during rainstorms, and are there leaks that
  need to be fixed?

• Does the water heater leak?

• Is the clothes dryer vented outdoors?

• Do you store furnishings or old books in the basement?

Laundry Room

• Are carpets vacuumed frequently and cleaned regularly?

• Do you have concrete floors under carpeting?

• Do you have upholstered furniture that can harbor dust mites?

• Is there visible mold on window and door frames and ledges?

• Do you have an air conditioning unit that may be harboring mold?

• Are there leaks in the room that contribute to dampness
  and mold growth?

• Do you have houseplants in the room?

• During pollen season, are windows left open, allowing pollen
  to enter the room?

• Are there damp areas that are harboring mold?

• Does flooding occur during rainstorms, and are there leaks that
  need to be fixed?

• Does the water heater leak?

• Is the clothes dryer vented outdoors?

Working with Your Doctor

Without question, the best way to manage your reactions to indoor allergens is through avoidance. If you don't come into contact with the allergens that trigger your reactions, you won't develop symptoms. Avoiding indoor allergens is usually easier than avoiding outdoor ones. By taking the steps outlined in this chapter, you should be able to greatly reduce your exposure to the offenders within your home and work environments.

Nevertheless, it is not always possible to eliminate the offending allergens completely. If this is the case for you, your doctor can recommend medications that can significantly reduce the severity of your symptoms or may even prevent their onset. A complete description of the medications used to prevent and treat allergic reactions (including allergy shots) can be found in Chapter 5, along with a discussion of when and how they should be used.

You can help your physician determine the precise nature of your problem with indoor allergens by completing the questionnaire on the following pages and sharing this information at the time of your next doctor's visit. Complete the questionnaire now, and bring this book (or a copy of the completed questionnaire) with you to your next appointment.

SYMPTOM RESPONSE CHART

Before I took steps to minimize my reaction to indoor allergens, my symptoms were:

Symptom	**Severity*** **(before changes)**
runny nose	_____
sneezing	_____
itchy nose	_____
postnasal drip	_____
nasal congestion	_____
cough	_____
itchy, watery eyes	_____
headaches	_____
fatigue	_____
other (_____)	_____

I have taken the following steps to eliminate allergens in my home:

_____

_____

_____

_____

_____

_____

_____

SYMPTOM RESPONSE CHART

After I implemented the indoor allergy-fighting strategies, my symptoms changed in the following way:

Symptom	Severity* (after changes)
runny nose	_____
sneezing	_____
itchy nose	_____
postnasal drip	_____
nasal congestion	_____
cough	_____
itchy, watery eyes	_____
headaches	_____
fatigue	_____
other (_____)	_____

*Severity Scale (0-3 Scale):

0 = none

1 = mild

2 = moderate

3 = severe

Chapter 4

Making the Diagnosis of Allergy

M any people suffer from allergic symptoms simply because their
problem is never correctly diagnosed as an allergy. Others
know they have allergies, but are unable to control the problem
because they never identify the specific allergens that are causing
them to react. That's why an accurate diagnosis is so critical. To
insure that an accurate diagnosis is made, your doctor will need to
complete the first two of the following three steps, and then, if necessary, proceed to the third:

> • A complete medical history
> • A thorough physical examination
> • Appropriate diagnostic testing

The Medical History

Allergy specialists say that the overwhelming majority of allergy problems can be diagnosed — or at least strongly suspected — on the basis

of the medical history alone. It's not difficult to diagnose a food allergy in people who have severe reactions every time they eat peanuts, nor is it hard to determine that people who have severe nasal congestion and itchy, watery eyes throughout every spring are most likely allergic to pollens. And people who can breathe clearly at home, but become totally "stuffed up" when visiting friends with cats, usually suspect that they are allergic to the pets.

But not all allergies are that easy to diagnose, and not all allergens are that obvious. That's why your physician will need to take a detailed history, not only asking general medical questions, but also covering many areas that deal specifically with allergies and allergy symptoms.

The specific allergy-related questions your physician will need to ask include the following:

Family History

   • Do your parents have allergies?
This question helps the doctor determine if you are at high or low risk for allergies. If neither of your parents has an allergy, your risk of having one is about 15 - 25%; if one of your parents has an allergy, your risk of allergy goes up to about 30 - 50%; if both have allergies, your risk rises to about 60 - 75%.

Past Allergy History

   • Have you been diagnosed with allergies before?
   • If so, when?
   • What symptoms did you experience?
   • What allergens were identified?

- How often did the symptoms occur?
- How long did they last?
- Did any complications result (sinusitis, ear infection, asthma)?
- What tests were done (if any) to confirm the diagnosis?
- How were you treated?
- How did you respond to the treatment?
- What did you do to reduce your exposure to the responsible allergens?
- How successful were you at avoiding them?

Your answers to these questions will enable your physician to determine the severity of your illness and to decide whether it is necessary to perform or repeat certain diagnostic tests.

Current Allergy Status

- Are you having any allergy symptoms at this time?
- What are they?
- When do they occur?
- What makes them worse?
- What makes them improve?
- Are you taking any medication for allergies?
- If so, which one(s)? How often? In what dosage?
- Have you used other allergy medications in the past? Which ones?

Your answers to these questions will help the doctor determine whether your current symptoms are due to an allergy or some other kind of medical problem (see box: *Is It An Allergy Or A Cold?*). If all signs point to an allergy, your answers will help the doctor decide if additional life-style changes (for allergen avoidance) might help you, or whether it is appropriate to initiate medical therapy now. If the use of medication is deemed advisable, your past experience with drugs will help the doctor determine which ones are most likely to produce relief at this time.

If you are visiting a doctor for the first time because of a problem with allergies, you can expect to be asked all of these questions—and more. You will find a typical allergy history questionnaire in Chapter 12 on pages 230-232. Before you visit the doctor, you should prepare written answers to all of the questions in it. This will help you to answer the questions completely and accurately, and it will save a great deal of time that can be used to cover other issues during your visit.

IS IT AN ALLERGY OR A COLD?

Symptom	Allergy	Cold or Infection
Nasal discharge	Clear, thin & watery	Clear, changing to thick, yellow/green
Fever	No	Low-grade
Muscle aches	No	Often
Itching	Ears, nose & throat	Rarely
Sneezing	Common in "spells"	Sometimes
Duration	Weeks to months	7 to 10 days
Seasonal	Often	Mostly fall, winter

Reprinted with permission of The Asthma & Allergy Foundation of America.

The Physical Examination

After reviewing your medical history, the doctor will perform a complete medical examination, with special attention paid to your eyes, nose, ears, throat and skin. (If you have already had a general physical exam by another physician, your allergy examination may be limited to the particular areas related to your symptoms.) Typically, the "allergy exam" will include an examination of the inside of the nose for signs of inflammation, swelling and discoloration; the ears for signs of fluid in the middle ear; the lungs for signs of asthma; and the skin for evidence of allergic reactions.

Diagnostic Tests

Depending on your medical history and what is found on physical examination, your doctor may order tests that can confirm the general diagnosis of allergy and identify the specific allergens that are causing your reactions. In addition, the doctor may order other tests to be sure that a different type of medical problem is not causing your symptoms. For example, in a person with severe, persistent nasal congestion, thyroid function tests or a sinus x-ray might be ordered because hypothyroidism or sinusitis can also cause this condition.

Among the specific allergy tests your physician might order are the following:

Skin Test

What is it? The skin test is the gold standard of allergy diagnosis. The allergy specialist or a member of his or her team places diluted liquid—derived from allergens themselves—on the skin. It can confirm whether you have allergies, and determine what you are allergic to (pollen, dust mites, mold, pets, foods). It may also suggest the degree of your sensitivity.

How is it done? A drop of the suspected allergen is placed on the skin, then the skin is punctured or scratched with a needle or another device. Sometimes the allergen is first placed on the prongs of the device, so it is introduced at the same time the skin is punctured. Within fifteen minutes, if a skin reaction occurs that looks like a mosquito bite (for example, a red, raised, itchy welt or hive), the test has detected IgE (immunoglobulin E) specific to that allergen.

What are its advantages/disadvantages? When a large number of different allergens are being tested for, you will have to endure a prick or puncture for each of them — sometimes 40 or more separate pricks in a single session. As unpleasant as that sounds, it is really not very painful, and it is a particularly effective and reproducible technique for diagnosing sensitivities to pollen, dust mites, mold spores and animal dander. The results are available in about 15 minutes.

Special considerations. If you've been taking antihistamine medications or some antidepressants, you may need to stop using them for at least three days (sometimes more) before the skin test is performed. Be sure to advise your doctor of all medications you are taking.

RAST

What is it? RAST, or radioallergosorbent testing, is a blood test that can diagnose the presence of allergies.

How is it done? The test involves drawing a blood sample, which is sent to a laboratory where an allergen is added to it. Using a technique called radioimmunoassay, the blood is then evaluated for the presence of IgE antibodies against this allergen.

What are its advantages/disadvantages? With RAST, tests involving many allergens can be performed on a single blood sample, and thus it requires just one needle stick even in the case of multiple allergen testing.

RAST, however, is not as sensitive as skin tests, and it may miss diagnosing some allergies. It also is more costly. Nevertheless, it may be advisable for very young children for whom skin testing may be difficult. It is also a good choice for people who are currently taking medication that interferes with skin tests (particularly those who cannot stop the medication for a few days), and for those who cannot tolerate skin tests due to extensive eczema or other skin rashes.

Special considerations. Be prepared to wait about five to seven days or more for the results of RAST.

Nasal Smear

What is it? This procedure examines cells in the nasal discharge of a patient suspected of having allergies.

How is it done? Secretions are taken from the nose, typically by scraping with a flexible plastic probe. The secretions are then put on a slide and examined under the microscope. Specifically, levels of white blood cells called eosinophils are counted; these cells tend to accumulate in greater numbers in the nasal passages of people with allergies.

What are its advantages/disadvantages? The nasal smear test is a low-cost technique that can help in the diagnosis of allergic rhinitis. However, it is not considered a definitive diagnostic test, and at times the test is negative even if the person is allergic. Nevertheless, the test findings can be used to support the diagnosis of allergic rhinitis and to differentiate this condition from a cold.

Chapter 5

Treating Your Allergies with Medications

Avoidance of allergens is always the best way to prevent allergic reactions and the symptoms that accompany them, but complete avoidance can be very difficult. When the winds blow in the spring, pollens are everywhere — including the air you'll be forced to breathe if you step outdoors. And allergen avoidance is almost impossible for some people, like letter carriers, gardeners and construction workers, whose jobs force them to be in contact with airborne allergens. In all of these situations, the proper use of medication can eliminate the misery that usually accompanies the allergic reactions and greatly improve one's quality of life.

Allergy drugs can be used for prevention (to block an allergic reaction before it gets started or to keep it from progressing) or to relieve symptoms after an allergic reaction has started. Some allergy drugs are designed for only one of these purposes; others, however, can be used to accomplish both goals.

Several different types of drugs can be used to treat allergies, and they differ greatly in the way they work in the body. The key to success with all of them depends on taking them according to your doctor's directions. If taken early enough, some of these drugs may actually prevent the allergic reaction from starting. Others will halt the reaction before it can progress to the point where symptom-causing chemicals are released. As doctors have found, there are several different points at which drugs can interfere with the allergic process and prevent or minimize the development of symptoms:

- Drugs may stabilize the mast cells, so they are less likely to release chemicals, like histamine, that initiate the allergic reaction and cause inflammation in the nose and respiratory passages.

- Drugs may block the attachment of symptom-causing chemicals, like histamine, to cell receptors. The most troublesome physical changes caused by histamine won't take place if it cannot attach to cells.

- Drugs may reverse or prevent the inflammation that can follow an allergic reaction. (If the inflammation is not treated, the symptoms will persist even if the allergic process is not ongoing.)

Using Drugs for Relief. Several different types of drugs (sometimes called *rescue* medications) can be used to provide symptomatic relief of allergy symptoms, although they do not affect the underlying disease process. These drugs are appropriate when the allergic response is underway, because they will provide temporary relief and comfort. However, something will need to be done to address the underlying allergic reaction that is causing the symptoms, because these drugs do not offer a long-term solution to the problem. There are several different ways these rescue drugs work:

- Some drugs constrict (narrow) blood vessels in the mucous membranes of the nose, which reduces the amount of blood flowing to the area. This in turn helps to "shrink" the swollen tissues in the nose, reduces inflammation, decreases mucus production, relieves congestion and makes it easier to breathe through the nose.

- Some drugs help block late phases of the inflammatory response, thus reducing the number of cells that release symptom-causing chemicals, easing local irritation and swelling, and decreasing nasal secretions.

When the allergic process is already underway and has progressed to the point where symptoms are present, it is usually necessary to use both *rescue* and *preventive* types of medications. The *rescue* drugs will provide temporary relief of symptoms while the *preventive* medications suppress the allergic reaction and reverse the inflammation that has already occurred.

Here are the general categories of medications used to care for allergies:

- **Antihistamines** interfere with the process by which chemicals —specifically, histamine—attach themselves to cells and set an allergic reaction into motion. Remember, allergy symptoms occur because histamine attaches itself to "histamine receptors" on other cells—almost like a key would be inserted into a lock. If the histamine attaches to these receptors, the door is opened for the reaction that produces the discomforting symptoms. Antihistamines, however, work by attaching to the receptor sites before histamine can get to them, leaving no room at those sites for histamine. The allergic reaction is disrupted because the antihistamines — though able to attach to the same receptors — do

OVER-THE-COUNTER (NONPRESCRIPTION) DRUGS

Once your doctor has diagnosed you as having allergies, he or she may recommend trying an over-the-counter allergy medication as a first step in your treatment. Theses OTC drugs tend to be less expensive than prescription medications, but like all drugs, they may cause side effects. All over-the-counter antihistamines, for example, may cause drowsiness.

Studies show that between 25-50% of those who use nonprescription antihistamines will experience side effects (see page 87).

For those who experience sedation or other side effects with nonprescription antihistamines, newer prescription drugs may be a better alternative. The side-effects profile of these medications differs from that of OTC antihistamines. Most of these drugs do not cause sedation.

Your doctor can play a role in the decision about which drugs to choose. He or she can not only select an appropriate medication for you, but also can help monitor its side effects.

not trigger the same harmful changes as histamine. They may begin to provide relief in one hour.

- **Decongestants** constrict small arteries, thus decreasing the amount of blood flowing through them. This, in turn, reduces the leakage of fluids from blood vessels that occurs during an allergic reaction. Decongestants are particularly effective for relieving the symptoms of nasal stuffiness. They also contract large veins in the nose, thereby reducing swelling and making breathing easier.

- **Mast cell stabilizers** interfere with the release of histamine by mast cells after a sensitized person is exposed to an allergen. This helps to prevent or reduce inflammation in those tissues. If used properly, mast cell stabilizers can be quite effective at preventing or minimizing nasal allergy symptoms, including congestion.

- **Corticosteroids** are hormonal medications that manage the inflammation that accompanies a persistent allergic reaction. These drugs are particularly effective for patients with chronic nasal allergies. They reduce mucus production and cut down on nasal congestion.

- **Anticholinergics** work by blocking the effect of acetylcholine, a chemical that helps the nervous system transmit messages, including messages that cause the secretion of mucus in the nose and respiratory passages. After an allergic reaction affecting these sites, the irritation that follows can trigger acetylcholine to excessively stimulate the mucus-secreting glands. In some patients, anticholinergic medication is an effective way to dry up a runny nose.

In the pages that follow, you will find more detailed information about the drugs described above and how they can help you manage your allergies.

Antihistamines

Many physicians consider antihistamines to be the first line of therapy for people with mild or intermittent allergic symptoms. If your allergy symptoms include a runny nose, sneezing and itchy, watery eyes, you should be able to get relief with an antihistamine. These drugs help dry out the nasal membranes, and may begin relieving symptoms in some patients as soon as 30 minutes after taking them.

However, they will not open up a congested nose. Antihistamines should be taken as directed by your doctor.

Side Effects of Antihistamines

The first-generation antihistamines are able to penetrate into the central nervous system. As a result, they generally cause more side effects than the newer, second-generation prescription drugs. In 25 - 50% of patients, the older drugs cause side effects such as drowsiness, nervousness, constipation, dry mouth and difficulty urinating. Many people are unaware of how much the sedating antihistamines can interfere with daily life. In fact, these drugs carry warnings regarding driving a car or operating machinery. (Pilots are prohibited by law from using sedating antihistamines for at least 24 hours before a flight.)

Antihistamines have been available for decades in pill and liquid form. In 1997, the first antihistamine nasal spray became available by prescription.

Nonprescription antihistamines, all of which fall into the sedating category, are relatively inexpensive. There are literally hundreds of products from which to choose, but many are simply different brand names for the same small group of drugs that have been available for many years. Among the most easily recognized names are Benadryl® (diphenhydramine), Chlor-Trimeton® (chlorpheniramine), Tavist-1® (clemastine) and Dimetapp® (brompheniramine).

Nonsedating antihistamines, available only by prescription, may be appropriate if you need to stay mentally alert, or perform complex tasks such as driving a car or operating machinery.

Aside from sedation, serious side effects are rare with both prescription and nonprescription antihistamines *when they are taken according to manufacturers' instructions* (some antihistamines should be used only once a day; others require more frequent dosing). However, when taken in high doses, antihistamines can cause heart palpitations or a rapid heartbeat. Also, people who have narrow-angle glaucoma and men who have prostate enlargement should not take first-generation antihistamines except under the supervision of a physician. The safety of antihistamines during pregnancy has not been established; pregnant women should consult their physicians before taking antihistamines.

One important warning: Prescription antihistamines terfenadine (Seldane®—no longer available in the U.S.) and astemizole (sold under the brand name Hismanal®) can have a potentially fatal side effect (abnormal heart rhythm) if taken in combination with a number of drugs, including certain antifungal agents, antibiotics or other drugs. **These cases are very rare, but it is essential that these drug**

WHEN SHOULD YOU USE A COMBINATION MEDICATION?

Though both antihistamines and decongestants have allergy-fighting properties, neither can manage *all* of your allergy symptoms. That's why doctors often recommend the use of both drugs at the same time. For the sake of convenience, some pharmaceutical companies have combined both types of drugs into a single pill or syrup. Many allergists consider this popular one-two punch to be a more effective medication for relieving the symptoms of allergic rhinitis than either drug alone. Several such combination drugs are now available, in both over-the-counter and prescription products. Most need to be taken 2-4 times a day, but once-a-day formulations are available.

combinations be avoided. Be sure to tell your physician about all the drugs you are taking.

The Bottom Line on Antihistamines

If an over-the-counter antihistamine relieves your symptoms, and you're *not* bothered by grogginess or other side effects when taking nonprescription antihistamines, you and your physician may decide that they are an appropriate choice for you. If they don't work, or if side effects are a problem, discuss the prescription antihistamines with your doctor to determine if one of them would be more appropriate in your particular case. Remember, drowsiness can sneak up on you and slow you down, so see your doctor if you have any questions about your medications.

Decongestants

While antihistamines can control many rhinitis symptoms, they are not very effective for treating nasal stuffiness once it has developed. That's where decongestants can help. They provide relief by constricting dilated blood vessels, thus reducing blood flow to the nasal region, shrinking swollen membranes, opening up congested nasal passages and making breathing easier. However, they cannot alleviate many of the other symptoms of allergic rhinitis, such as sneezing, itching and watery eyes.

Decongestants are available in tablet or liquid form, as well as in eye and nose drops and sprays; many are over-the-counter, but some require a prescription. All forms of decongestants are effective, although nasal sprays tend to work more rapidly (often within seconds).

Side Effects of Decongestants

Oral decongestants can stimulate the central nervous system and trigger irritability, nervousness, headaches, insomnia, increased blood pressure and a rapid heartbeat. And, because they constrict blood vessels throughout the body, they may raise blood pressure and/or increase the heart rate in some people. For this reason, it's a good idea to talk to your doctor before using oral decongestants and then to take only the recommended doses. Prescription decongestants are also available which may have different side effects.

Adverse effects are infrequent with decongestant nasal sprays (such as Afrin® and Neo-Synephrine®), but people do sometimes complain of sneezing and dryness with them. Prolonged use of decongestant sprays must be avoided, because of the "rebound" effect this can produce. Chronic use causes the mucous membranes in the nose to become irritated and inflamed, and allergy symptoms — particularly nasal stuffiness — can actually become *worse* than before the drug was started. Doctors call this rebound condition "rhinitis medicamentosa" (medicine-induced rhinitis).

Ironically, when rebound stuffiness occurs, many people increase their use of the nasal sprays, convinced that they need *more* to resolve their symptoms. A vicious cycle begins, and many of these allergy sufferers become virtually "addicted" to their spray medications. Some people experience rebound stuffiness after using nasal sprays for just three to four days. If congestion persists for more than a few days while using these medications, the spray should be discontinued and the use of oral decongestants (pills or liquid) or other treatments should be discussed with your doctor.

The Bottom Line on Decongestants

Spray decongestants should only be used occasionally for relief of nasal congestion, not in an ongoing way as a preventive measure. Decongestants can combat an allergy episode as it occurs and should be taken as soon as your nose becomes congested. If treatment is needed for more than a few days, oral decongestants are a better choice than nasal sprays.

Cromolyn Sodium (Mast Cell Stabilizers)

In 1997, an anti-inflammatory nasal spray, cromolyn sodium, previously available only by prescription, became available over-the-counter.

Cromolyn sodium is a so-called mast cell stabilizer; it works by inhibiting the release of histamine, which, in turn, reduces inflammation in the nasal passages. Cromolyn sodium can also be used to prevent or treat allergy symptoms such as a runny nose, sneezing, and nasal itching and stuffiness, but results are not rapid.

Proper use of cromolyn sodium requires persistence and patience. One to four weeks of use (one spray per nostril every four to six hours) are required for relief of symptoms. When taken prophylactically, the dosage is the same.

Side Effects of Cromolyn

A small percentage of people using cromolyn sodium have complained of stinging and dryness in their nostrils, sneezing and headaches, but these side effects are only temporary. The drug does not cause drowsiness or any other significant adverse effects, including rebound congestion.

The Bottom Line on Cromolyn

For best results when taking cromolyn sodium prophylactically, regular use should start at least one to two weeks *before* the beginning of "hay fever" season, and continue throughout the pollen season. Good to excellent results have been achieved by patients who follow this recommendation. However, cromolyn needs to be taken four or more times a day for maximum effectiveness, a schedule that many people find very difficult to maintain.

Nasal Steroid Sprays

Different physicians prefer different treatment options. Another alternative for controlling the distressing symptoms of allergic rhinitis is the use of corticosteroid sprays, which are available only by prescription. These sprays contain potent anti-inflammatory hormones, which some physicians believe are the most effective drugs for managing allergic rhinitis.

Corticosteroids work by suppressing inflammation in the nasal membranes, reducing the number of mast cells and eosinophils, and decreasing the production of mucus. This clears the nasal passages for easier breathing. However, because nasal steroid sprays do not relieve itchy eyes and palate, some people who choose this alternative may also need to take an antihistamine or use eye drops.

Some nasal steroid products use wet sprays; others deliver a pressurized aerosol. Depending on the doctor's choice, the pharmacist will

HOW TO USE YOUR STEROID SPRAY OR INHALER

Always follow the directions on the prescription insert.

1. Clear your nasal passages by gently blowing your nose into a handkerchief or tissue.

2. Wash your hands with soap and water.

3. Shake the drug container, and remove its cap.

4. Press an index finger on one nostril, closing it off. Keep your mouth closed.

5. Place the tip of the inhaler or spray into the open nostril, pointing it away from the nasal septum.

6. Activate the container by squeezing or pumping it. At the same time, inhale deeply through the open nostril.

7. Hold your breath for several seconds, and then exhale through your mouth.

8. Repeat steps 4 through 7 with the other nostril (unless your doctor has instructed you to administer the drug through only one nostril).

9. Place the cap back on the container.

dispense either a mechanical pump spray mister or a metered-dose inhaler to administer the drug. It is critical that these devices be used correctly to ensure that the steroids actually reach the tissues they are intended to treat (see box above).

When steroid sprays are used to treat symptoms, most people will require one or two squirts or puffs per nostril, administered one to two times a day. Once symptoms are under control, it may be possible to cut back to once-a-day dosing, which is the lowest dose that can provide control and prevent further outbreaks.

Side Effects of Steroid Sprays

When used appropriately, nasal steroid sprays infrequently cause side effects. Some patients experience dryness, itching or burning in the nasal passages, as well as sneezing, but these responses can be reduced if the spray device is used properly. Steroid sprays are a safer alternative than oral corticosteroid drugs (see box on next page).

The Bottom Line on Steroid Sprays

It may take several days for nasal steroids to begin to manage allergy symptoms, although the full effects may not be felt for two to three weeks. This medication needs time to suppress any inflammation that is present in the nose before airborne allergens can trigger allergic reactions. For maximum benefit, nasal steroids should be taken daily. If treatment is stopped during allergy season, symptoms may recur within just a few days.

Anticholinergic Medication

Ipratropium bromide, a nasal spray that works at the site of chemical receptors in the nose, is the first anticholinergic drug available by prescription for allergies. It prevents acetylcholine, a neurotransmitter that stimulates the production of mucus, from attaching to these receptors, thus decreasing the production of mucus.

Ipratropium is administered in a dose of one to two sprays per nostril per day. It can relieve a runny nose but has no effect on congestion, sneezing or an itchy nose.

Side Effects of Anticholinergic Medications

Anticholinergic medications have minimal side effects (most commonly, nasal dryness and nose bleeding), and these occur rarely.

STEROIDS: HOW BIG A RISK?

Some people are reluctant to use any steroid drugs because of stories they've heard about serious side effects. In fact, most of these adverse effects have occurred when anabolic sex steroids have been abused by people who were trying to build up their muscle mass for athletic purposes, or when high doses of corticosteroids have been taken for long periods of time.

The corticosteroids used to treat allergic rhinitis are a completely different type of medication from the anabolic sex steroids. Also, the doses used in nasal sprays and inhalers are minute compared to the high doses of oral steroids that have led to complications in the past. By delivering the spray directly to the nasal tissues that require treatment, it is possible to obtain dramatic relief with very low doses that do not affect other parts of the body. Nasal steroids are safe and effective when used properly.

Even though corticosteroids are available in pill form, these tablets do not play a major role in treating allergic rhinitis, primarily because serious side effects can result if they are used regularly over long periods of time. However, in people who have severe nasal rhinitis that has not improved after treatment with other medications such as antihistamines and decongestants, a short course (about three to five days) of treatment with oral steroids may occasionally be appropriate.

Nevertheless, anticholinergics are not recommended for people with narrow-angle glaucoma or an enlarged prostate.

The Bottom Line on Anticholinergic Medications

If an allergy-related runny nose is the only symptom you have, ipratropium may be appropriate to use. However, anticholinergics cannot relieve symptoms such as sneezing and nasal congestion. Some doctors may also prescribe anticholinergics as an adjunct to other drugs— for example, to relieve a runny nose—while steroids are managing the underlying inflammation.

Strategies for Medication Use

To get the most out of your allergy medications, you need to take them correctly. Here are some guidelines to keep in mind:

• Before you leave the doctor's office, make sure you understand precisely how much medication you should be taking, and how frequently it should be taken. Be certain that these instructions agree with the label that your pharmacist affixes to the drug container. Do not waver from the dosage guidelines without consulting your physician.

• For over-the-counter medications, follow the label instructions carefully. Be aware that dosages for younger children (according to their age or weight) are typically lower than they are for adults.

• If you experience side effects that disrupt day-to-day living or you have concern about them, call your doctor, who should be able to adjust the dosage or switch you to a different medication (for example, from a sedating antihistamine to a nonsedating one). Since allergy medications may need to be taken for years, be sure to discuss both the short- and long-term effects of all drugs you are using with your doctor and your pharmacist.

- Inform your doctor if you are considering stopping the use of birth control and planning to become pregnant. To ensure the safety of both mother and fetus, it may be necessary to change the allergy drugs that are used during pregnancy.

- Discard any drug whose expiration date has passed.

Can Allergy Shots Help?

If allergy medications and/or environmental controls don't put a halt to your sneezing and drippy nose, where can you turn? Your doctor may recommend allergy shots. Physicians use the terms *immuno-therapy* and *hyposensitization* to describe this treatment, and although it works for many people, it's certainly not an overnight cure. In fact, it usually requires frequent visits to the doctor's office over a period of several years.

SPRAYS, NOT SHOTS?

If you cringe at the thought of all of those needles that are part of immunotherapy, there may soon be a less painful alternative. Recent research shows that immunotherapy might someday be given as a nasal spray. These studies found that nasal administration may be particularly effective in people with allergies to dust mites or pollen. Other research has been aimed at reducing the number of immunotherapy injections, even exploring the possibility of limiting the course of treatment to just eight weeks.

Immunotherapy involves injections of the very allergen to which you're allergic. With each shot, the concentration of the allergen is increased slightly. Over time, this allows the body to gradually build tolerance to the allergen, so the immune system stops reacting to the harmless substance. This, in turn, prevents the release of histamine and other allergy-related substances.

Keep in mind that allergy shots that are part of immunotherapy are different than those that you get to protect you from the measles, hepatitis or influenza. Immunotherapy shots are custom-made for each patient, containing liquid-based extracts of the precise substances (for example, dust mites, weed pollen, animal dander) that you're allergic to, typically based on the findings of the diagnostic tests (skin tests, RAST testing) that your physician has already conducted.

In a typical immunotherapy scenario, the patient initially receives shots on a weekly basis (sometimes more often). Over time, the frequency of treatment gradually decreases to once a month. The shots may be required for as long as three to five years, although the first noticeable improvements in allergy symptoms usually begin in about three to six months. About 65% of patients who receive immunotherapy experience some degree of relief from their symptoms for many years after the injections have ended. However, some individuals may need to resume therapy after the three- to five-year time frame if symptoms gradually reappear; some may never be able to stop taking the shots.

Side Effects of Immunotherapy

Most people tolerate immunotherapy very well, although some will develop moderate swelling and redness at the site of the injections.

YOUR MEDICATION SCHEDULE

Use the chart below to record the medication regimen that your doctor has prescribed.

Medication	Dose	Frequency
_____	_____	_____
_____	_____	_____
_____	_____	_____
_____	_____	_____
_____	_____	_____
_____	_____	_____
_____	_____	_____
_____	_____	_____
_____	_____	_____
_____	_____	_____
_____	_____	_____
_____	_____	_____
_____	_____	_____
_____	_____	_____
_____	_____	_____
_____	_____	_____

Occasionally, people experience systemic reactions to the shots, with symptoms such as itchy eyes, sneezing, nasal drip, swelling of the throat, chest tightness, cough and dizziness. These types of reactions occur in only one out of every 1,000 (or more) injections. To be safe, patients are asked to remain in the doctor's office for 20 to 30 minutes after the shots are given to ensure that serious adverse effects, if they occur, will take place under medical supervision. There is an increased risk with immunotherapy for people who have coronary heart disease and are taking beta-blocker medications for it, those with severe atopic dermatitis or severe asthma, and those having increased allergy symptoms on the day of the immunotherapy shot.

The Bottom Line on Immunotherapy

People with seasonal allergies only (during "hay fever" season, for example) get better results with immunotherapy than those with perennial (year-round) allergic rhinitis. If avoidance strategies and treatments with medications fail to sufficiently relieve allergy symptoms, immunotherapy is an appropriate additional treatment to consider.

Chapter 6

Food Allergies

About 25% of Americans believe they are allergic to certain foods
because they have bad reactions after eating those foods. Most
people have a tendency to lump all bad food reactions together and
assume that they're "allergic" to any food that induces a reaction. In
fact, most food-related reactions have nothing to do with *allergy* or
the immune system. They are the result of other adverse food reactions, commonly referred to as food *intolerance*. Scientific studies
show that true food allergies affect only 3 - 6% of children under the
age of three and only 1 - 2% of adults.

Although the symptoms of both food allergy and food intolerance
often seem similar, there's a big difference in the underlying processes that produce these symptoms:

- In people with food allergies, reactions occur because their
  immune system reacts inappropriately and produces IgE antibodies against a harmless substance in the food (usually a protein). Each time that food is eaten, a reaction is triggered, causing the release of histamine and other chemicals, which causes
  allergic symptoms to occur.

- In people with food intolerance, the immune system is not

involved and antibodies are not produced. The recurrent symptoms are produced instead by one or more of the following mechanisms.

Causes of Food Intolerance

- **Pharmacologic sensitivity:** This is a predictable reaction to a chemical in the food. The extent of the reaction is influenced by the amount of chemical consumed and the individual's degree of sensitivity to the chemical. Caffeine is a perfect example of such a chemical. Almost anyone will be kept awake by drinking several cups of coffee before bedtime. But some people are able to consume moderate amounts of caffeine during the day, without any adverse reaction, while others get jittery after just a few sips of coffee or a cola drink.

- **Chemical sensitivity:** This is an unpredictable reaction that causes some people to have severe symptoms after consuming food containing a specific chemical, while others can consume large amounts without reacting at all. Examples of such chemicals and some of the reactions they produce include: tyramine (found in aged cheeses and red wines), which can trigger migraine headaches in some people; MSG (a flavor enhancer commonly used in Asian restaurants), which causes headaches or chest pain in sensitive individuals; and sulfites (used to prevent mold growth in wines, beer and dried fruit), which can trigger allergic reactions, including anaphylaxis and asthmatic episodes, in some people.

- **Enzyme deficiencies:** These reactions are caused by deficiencies in enzymes that the body requires to digest and process foods normally in the gastrointestinal tract. The most common deficiency involves lactase, an enzyme required for the digestion of lactose, a sugar found naturally in milk. People with lactase deficiency develop nausea, bloating, cramping and gas if they consume excessive amounts of milk or certain other dairy products. Several options are available to such individuals. Most people who are intolerant to lactose can reduce or eliminate their symptoms if they use dairy products that have been pretreated with lactase enzyme or if they eat smaller portions.

- **Other physical disorders:** Many physical disorders can cause recurrent symptoms after eating by interfering with the digestion of foods or with the flow of foods through the intestinal tract. For example, hiatal hernia and gastroesophageal reflux disease (GERD) cause regurgitation of food and acid from the stomach into the esophagus; gall bladder disease makes some people intolerant to fatty foods.

- **Physiologic reactions:** Some people mistakenly believe they are allergic to certain foods when they are, in fact, having the same kind of normal or "physiologic" reactions and symptoms that most people would experience after eating those foods. A good example of this is the gassiness that follows the consumption of foods like beans or cabbage. Many people also develop mild food intolerances as they age. For reasons that are not completely understood, foods that were once easily tolerated begin to cause mild intestinal "upsets" as people get older.

- **Food "poisoning":** Some reactions erroneously blamed on food allergy are actually the result of toxic substances in food or contamination of food by bacteria and viruses. This is usually easy to distinguish from allergic food reactions because food poisoning occurs infrequently, the illness that follows is usually short-lived, and it does not recur every time the particular food is eaten. Examples of this type of problem include the widespread — but short-lived— outbreaks of food poisoning that were due to contaminated hamburger meat and unpasteurized apple juice. As soon as the sources of contamination were eliminated, so were the problems.

• **Psychological reactions:** Occasionally, certain foods may trigger "psychological" reactions that can cause troublesome symptoms, even though there is no physical explanation— allergic or otherwise— for the problem. Included in this category are phobic reactions (in which case a fear of the food or something associated with the food triggers anxiety and other symptoms) and expectational reactions (symptoms arise because people expect a particular food to cause them distress— even though there is no chemical or physical reason for this to occur).

Foods that Cause Allergic Reactions

Almost any food can cause an allergic reaction, although most reactions are caused by foods that contain proteins (the allergenic part of the food is almost always a protein). A few foods, including shellfish, peanuts, tree nuts, eggs, wheat and milk, account for nearly 98% of all true food allergies.

The development of allergies to specific foods depends, in part, on the amount of exposure that people have to these foods. As a result, food allergies that are relatively common in one country or geographic location—where a particular food is extremely popular—

may occur much less often in a place where the food is rarely eaten. For example, a French study found that wheat, peanuts and crab were the most common cause of food allergies, while the foods most often implicated in a Spanish study were fruits and dried fruits. In the Spanish group, allergies to fish, eggs and cow's milk were very uncommon. The researchers who did this study attributed the unusual pattern to the typical dietary habits of the region in which the study was done.

In children, the foods that most frequently cause allergic reactions are milk, eggs, peanuts, wheat and soy, in that order. In adults, the most common foods to cause allergic reactions include peanuts (and other foods from the legume family), tree nuts (such as walnuts), fish and crustacean seafood (shrimp, prawns, crayfish, lobster and crab). Allergies to milk, eggs and wheat are less common in adults.

In addition, people may have food reactions caused by "cross-reactivity" with non-food allergens. This occurs when an allergen or antigen found in a food (typically a fruit or vegetable) is identical with or very similar to an allergen in a non-food source, such as pollen. For example, people who are sensitive to birch pollen may develop such cross-reactions within minutes after eating apples, carrots, parsnips, celery, hazelnuts, potatoes or kiwi. Some people who are allergic to tree and grass pollens may develop allergic symptoms after eating apples, tree nuts, peaches, oranges, pears, cherries, fennel, tomatoes or carrots.

Often, the symptoms that result from such cross-reactions are limited to the oral area, a condition known as "oral allergy syndrome." Itching of the mouth and lips is usually the most prominent symptom, although swelling of the lips, mouth and tongue can also occur, and the problem can become widespread.

FOOD ALLERGIES & ASTHMA

Can what you feed your child cause him or her to experience an asthmatic episode?

Yes, it's possible that food allergies can provoke asthmatic episodes in susceptible children. But even though it's true that allergies in general can trigger asthmatic episodes in both adults and children, food allergies play only a small role and tend to be much less of a problem than cats, dogs, dust mites or mold spores.

The Symptoms of Food Allergy

As with all allergic reactions, the primary symptoms of food allergy are caused by the release of histamine from mast cells that have been previously sensitized to specific food allergens. Whenever — and wherever — the sensitized mast cells come into contact with those allergens again, histamine release is likely to occur (this can happen within minutes of eating the food or as late as an hour afterwards). It is not surprising that the earliest and most common symptoms of food allergy, therefore, are related to the gastrointestinal tract.

Within minutes of eating a food to which you are allergic, the tissues of the mouth and throat may be affected, resulting in itching, tingling or swelling of the lips, tongue, roof of the mouth and throat. This may be accompanied by tightness in the throat, difficulty in speaking, and coughing. These uncomfortable symptoms may clear quickly without any further problems, or nausea, vomiting, cramps and diarrhea may develop as the offending food moves along through the gastrointestinal tract.

The body has some protective mechanisms for keeping food allergens inside the intestinal tract. When these mechanisms are working properly, all of the symptoms of food allergy will be limited to the gastrointestinal system. But, even though these protective mechanisms exist, a very small amount of allergens often get through the intestinal wall into the bloodstream, which then carries them to every organ in the body. When this happens, sensitized mast cells elsewhere in the body can come in contact with the allergens, triggering the release of histamine into the tissues of other organ systems.

When the histamine release occurs in the lungs, asthma episodes may be triggered. Histamine release in the nose and eyes will cause watering and congestion. And when histamine is released in the skin because of a food allergy, hives and swelling will result. Hives are probably the most common allergic food reaction outside the gastrointestinal system. In the most severe cases of food allergy, large enough amounts of histamine are released throughout the body to trigger a life-threatening anaphylactic reaction.

Making the Diagnosis: Is It a Food Allergy or Not?

Sometimes it is obvious when an allergy is responsible for adverse food reactions (for instance, when you develop immediate swelling of your lips and start wheezing every time you eat shrimp). In a case like this, it is still valuable to confirm the shrimp sensitivity with skin tests or a blood test (either RAST or an enzyme immune assay). Then you can take steps to prevent contact with the food. However, not all adverse food reactions are that easy to diagnose, because most of the tests available are not perfect.

The problem of diagnosing food allergy is complicated further by the fact that most of us consume literally hundreds of different food ingredients during the course of a typical week, and many of those ingredients are "hidden" in processed foods and home recipes. Was it the soy used to thicken a soup, the milk proteins in the baked goods, or the anchovies in the steak sauce that triggered the symptoms every time you used the product? Or was it the preservatives or the spices in these foods? Identifying the precise allergen causing your reactions can be tricky.

You and your physician will use the following key steps to determine whether a food allergy is causing your symptoms, and if so, which food is responsible:

- Medical history
- Physical examination
- Diet diaries
- Elimination diet
- Skin tests
- Blood tests
- Food challenge

Medical history: In many cases, a good medical history is the only thing needed to diagnose a food allergy. This is particularly true when an individual reacts in a typically allergic fashion (for example, with an itchy mouth and swollen tongue or by breaking out into hives) every time a particular food is eaten. Your doctor will pay special attention to the following key points in your history:

- **Family history:** Allergies tend to run in families. If one or both parents are or were allergic to anything (not necessarily to food), your risk of developing allergies yourself is increased (though you will not necessarily be allergic to the same thing as your parent). You should also tell your doctor if any other close relatives, such as grandparents or aunts and uncles, now have or have had allergies. One study found that peanut allergies are more common in the siblings of individuals with this same allergy, compared to their parents or the general population.

• **Personal history of allergy:** If you now have or have had any non-food allergic problems, you are at increased risk for also developing allergies to foods.

• **Consistent relationship between the consumption of a particular food and the pattern of symptoms:** When you are allergic to a food, similar symptoms should occur in approximately the same pattern every time you consume the food (although the severity of the symptoms may vary depending on the amount of food consumed). Other factors that can affect the nature and severity of the reaction include the following:

— The presence of other foods in the intestine tends to decrease the amount of allergen absorbed into the bloodstream, or at least slow its absorption.

— Increased stomach acidity tends to decrease the amount of allergen absorbed.

— Simultaneous ingestion of alcohol tends to increase the amount of allergen absorbed.

• **Nature of the reaction and symptoms:** Some symptoms and physical changes are highly suggestive of true allergy (such as itching of the lips, swelling of the tongue or hives) while others are more suggestive of nonallergic food intolerance (such as flushing, headache or chest pain).

Physical examination: Physical examination cannot be used alone to diagnose food allergy, but the exam may be helpful if it reveals changes that are typical of allergy, such as hives or eczema. The exam may also be useful if it helps the doctor identify a nonallergic condition that is causing you to have symptoms that can be confused with food allergy.

Food and symptom diaries: Sometimes it's difficult to make the connection between a particular food you are eating and the onset of symptoms. Most of us eat so many different foods — and so often on the run — it's impossible to keep track of everything, but a simple food and symptom diary can solve this problem.

The diary gives you and your doctor a chronological record of all the foods you have eaten and all the symptoms you have experienced. By keeping a diary for at least 14 days, you are more likely to detect a link between the consumption of a particular food and the onset of symptoms, especially if you eat the food several times while you are keeping the diary and the symptoms recur each time. If you are placed on an elimination diet later (see next page), the diary will provide your doctor with a "baseline" record of symptoms that can be compared to the symptom record you keep while on the elimination diet.

To make the diary useful, you must record every food you eat, the time you ate it, the amount you consumed, and the precise time, duration and nature of any adverse reactions you experience (even if they don't seem connected to a food you ate). If you eat packaged or processed foods, it's important to record the brand names, also, as your doctor may be aware of "hidden" ingredients or additives that could be triggering the reactions. It may also be helpful to save or copy food labels during the time you are keeping the diary, in case your doctor needs more information about the ingredients.

You will find an example of a food diary on pages 128-130. You may make photocopies of the diary if you need additional pages.

Elimination diet: One tool that can be helpful in diagnosing a food allergy is the *elimination diet.* This diet removes all traces of the most highly suspected foods from your daily food intake to see if your symptoms improve. (The elimination diet is practical only when one

MYTHS AND FACTS

Myth: People who are allergic to foods have a hard time finding anything they can safely eat.

Fact: While people with food allergies must avoid the foods that trigger their reactions, in most cases only one or two foods cause problems.

Myth: Children who are hypersensitive to sugar become hyperactive if they have any candy or sweets.

Fact: Studies have not proven that sugar can trigger any sensitivity reaction, including hyperactivity.

Myth: If your baby is allergic to cow's milk, he or she will never be able to eat any dairy products.

Fact: Many children outgrow their allergy to milk as their digestive system matures.

or two foods are suspected.) If your symptoms disappear completely after eliminating the suspected foods, you are *probably* allergic to
those foods, and simply avoiding them in the future should resolve
your problem. However, even if symptoms do disappear during an
elimination diet, the diagnosis of food allergy cannot be made with
certainty unless the symptoms recur upon re-introduction of the suspected food(s).

Before you start an elimination diet, your allergist will ask you to keep
a food diary for one or two weeks (see page 128). You will continue the
diary while on the elimination diet and compare the two records to see
if the frequency and/or severity of symptoms is really improving.

While on the elimination diet, it is very important to avoid the accidental consumption of the foods you are trying to eliminate. For
example, if eggs and peanuts are the foods you suspect of causing
allergic reactions, you've got to make sure that you don't consume
them as "hidden" ingredients in other foods. Eggs are hidden in
hundreds of foods, among them such popular items as mayonnaise,
many baked goods, cereals and soups; peanuts are commonly found in
cereals, chili, salsa, spaghetti sauce, gravies, pie crusts and a host of
other foods.

If three or more foods are suspected of triggering allergic reactions,
or if the simple elimination diet described on the previous page does
not succeed in identifying the foods that trigger your reactions, it may
be necessary to try a much more restricted diet. On this diet, most of
the foods you usually eat are temporarily eliminated, and your diet is
severely restricted to only very basic foods (either rice and water or a
hypoallergenic commercial preparation). Then, very gradually, other
foods are reintroduced one at a time into your diet to see if they cause

the return of symptoms. These severely restricted diets may require the help of a registered dietitian to ensure that the menu is tolerable and that your nutrition is adequate.

Skin tests: Skin tests are sometimes helpful in diagnosing a food allergy if specific "suspect" foods have already been identified or in identifying unsuspected foods for possible elimination or challenge. The skin tests indicate when IgE antibodies to a specific food are present. However, the tests are not 100% accurate. A positive skin test supports the diagnosis of food allergy but still does not guarantee that the symptoms are caused by the allergy. In fact, many people regularly eat foods to which they have tested positive without having any symptoms. A negative test does not completely rule out the possibility that allergy *is* the problem. The accuracy of skin tests for food allergies varies greatly with the particular food being tested. This is particularly true for fruits, vegetables and shellfish, where testing with fresh food may yield positive skin tests, while tests with commercial extracts are negative.

If you have had an anaphylactic reaction to a specific food in the past, your doctor may choose not to skin test you for this food, or may use a more diluted extract of the food for the skin test. Even with a diluted extract, a positive result on such a test contributes valuable information.

Keep in mind that skin test results are not reliable if you are using anti-histamine medications. When scheduling the test, advise your doctor of *all* medications, including both over-the-counter and prescription, that you are taking or have taken in the recent past. If you have been taking antihistamines only intermittently, stopping their use for 24 hours before the test should be sufficient; but if you have been using them regularly, you may need to wait three to seven days, depending on the drug. In the case of Hismanal®, you should stop using it one to three months before the test.

Blood tests: Blood tests offer another way to test for the presence of IgE antibodies against specific food allergens and are sometimes used to confirm the results of skin tests. Some physicians use blood tests instead of skin tests, because they can clearly demonstrate whether IgE antibodies to a specific food are present. Further, blood tests allow physicians to safely check for allergies after an anaphylactic reaction. Also, blood tests offer a simpler way to test children. However, blood tests are considerably more expensive, they are less sensitive than skin tests, and the results can vary from lab to lab. For this reason, skin tests are generally considered the preferred method. For more information about these diagnostic tests, see Chapter 4.

Food challenge: Another method for diagnosing food allergy — particularly if other tests have failed to make the diagnosis conclusively — is the food challenge. The food challenge can be done in what is called an "open" fashion, in which the suspected food is simply reintroduced into the diet to see if symptoms recur afterward. One problem with the open approach is that the individuals being challenged know they are consuming the suspected food, which can prejudice the results. The challenge is never done at home if there is a reason to believe that the person might have a severe reaction afterward.

The ultimate test for diagnosing a food allergy is the double-blind placebo-controlled food challenge (DBPCFC). In this test, small amounts of the suspected problem foods are packed into unlabeled, unscented gelatin capsules or some other vehicle. The patient is then asked to alternatively swallow these capsules and similar-appearing placebo capsules that contain only sugar or another hypoallergenic substance (the patient cannot tell which is which). The doctor then watches for any symptoms or physical reactions that follow the swallowing of each dose, as increasing amounts of food are given to the patient. To eliminate the possibility that the physician's observations are biased by knowing whether the patient is getting the food or the placebo, the challenge is done in a "double-blind" fashion. The capsules are coded by another member of the healthcare team and identified after the challenge is completed. During the test, the physician who observes the patient doesn't know which capsule the patient is receiving at any time.

Food challenges can successfully identify offending foods, but they are time-consuming and expensive. Because of the risk that an anaphylactic reaction could occur, these challenges must be done under a doctor's supervision in a medical facility equipped to handle such emergencies.

Unproven Methods for Diagnosing Food Allergies

Several scientifically unproven tests for food allergies are currently being offered to patients by a small number of practitioners. The primary danger in using these tests is that they can lead to the wrong diagnosis, which, in turn, leads to the wrong treatment. Also, they are very time-consuming and expensive. One of the most popular of these diagnostic tests for food allergy is cytotoxicity testing (also referred to as leukocytotoxic testing or Bryan's test). This test is done by mixing some of the patient's white blood cells with the suspected food antigens. Proponents of the test say that certain changes in the appearance of the blood cells indicate a "positive" test and an allergy to the food being evaluated. However, a number of well-controlled studies show that this test is not reproducible and is unreliable.

Another diagnostic test, called provocation-neutralization testing, involves giving the patient a small amount of allergen, either by injecting it under the skin or placing it under the tongue. The patient then reports any sensations that may arise during the next 10 minutes; if any occur, this is purportedly an indication of an allergy to the tested substance. The procedure is sometimes repeated with a higher dose if no reaction occurred the first time. However, there is no scientific evidence to support this method, and it involves considerable time and expense.

Avoidance: The Best Treatment

Once you have identified problem foods, the best (and only foolproof) way to prevent further reactions is to avoid eating those foods. This would be simple if you only ate single-ingredient, unprocessed foods. But it is difficult because the modern diet contains a wide variety of processed or manufactured foods, and these typically contain a large number of ingredients — many of which can trigger allergic reactions in sensitized individuals. These ingredients are often referred to as "hidden" allergens, because their presence is not obvious unless you carefully read the label (these hidden allergies may include milk proteins, eggs, texturizers, flavorings and emulsifiers). For a person with true and severe food allergies, even a small amount of these ingredients can turn an ordinarily "safe" food into an allergy trigger.

That's why if you have a food allergy, it's so important to carefully read ingredient labels every time you purchase a food product, even if the food is already familiar to you, and to be very cautious in restaurants. Manufacturers often produce new versions of old products, changing or adding ingredients in the process. If you have a food allergy, don't rely on your past success with a product to keep you safe. Check the label every time you purchase it again — just to be sure.

Be aware, also, that some listings on ingredient labels may refer to combinations of foods. For example, the term "modified food starch" can include a wide range of different source foods, including tapioca, potatoes, wheat, rice or corn. And the term "vegetable oils" can include a variety of different oil sources, including corn, safflower, sunflower and peanut oil.

At first, you may feel overwhelmed by how many ingredient labels you must read to keep from eating problem foods. Resources like The Food Allergy Network (see box on page 127) can help you.

Food Families

Just as animals are grouped into related groups (for example, crab, crayfish, lobster and shrimp are all crustaceans), plants and the foods they produce are grouped into related families. It is not unusual for animals and plants in the same "families" to share common protein allergens, and to cross-react with each other in laboratory tests. In spite of this strong similarity between foods in the same group, it is unusual for an allergic person to react to more than one food in a family. Still, such reactions can occur occasionally, so if you are allergic to one food in a plant or animal family, you should be cautious when eating other plants or animals in the same family.

The following list shows the major food families and their members:

Plant Sources

Apple family

Apple	Pear	Quince

Birch family

Filbert	Hazelnut

Buckwheat family

Buckwheat	Rhubarb

Gourd family

Cantaloupe	Honeydew melon	Pumpkin
Casaba	Muskmelon	Squash
Cucumber	Persian melon	Watermelon

Grain family

Barley	Gluten flour	Rice	Wheat germ
Bran	Graham flour	Rye	Wild rice
Cane	Malt	Sorghum	
Corn	Oats	Wheat	

Laurel family

Avocado	Bay leaf	Cinnamon

Legume family

Acacia	Lentil	Navy bean	Senna
Black-eyed pea	Licorice	Pea	String bean
Kidney bean	Lima bean	Peanut	Soybean

Lily family

Aloes	Chive	Leek
Asparagus	Garlic	Onion

Mustard family

Broccoli	Celery cabbage	Kohlrabi	Turnip
Brussels sprouts	Collard	Mustard	Watercress
Cabbage	Horseradish	Radish	
Cauliflower	Kale	Rutabaga	

Parsley family

Anise	Celery	Fennel
Caraway	Coriander	Parsley
Carrot	Dill	Parsnip

Plum family

Almond	Cherry	Peach	Prune
Apricot	Nectarine	Plum	

Potato family

Bell pepper	Green pepper	Red pepper`
Chili	Pimento	Tabasco
Eggplant	Potato	Tomato

Walnut family

Black walnut	English walnut	Pecan
Butternut	Hickory nut	

Animal Sources

Fish

Anchovy	Flounder	Pompano	Sunfish
Bass	Haddock	Salmon	Swordfish
Bluefish	Hake	Sardine	Trout
Carp	Halibut	Scrod	Tuna
Catfish	Herring	Shad	Weakfish
Codfish	Mackerel	Snapper	Whitefish
Drum	Mullet	Sole	
Eel	Pike	Sturgeon	

Fowl

Chicken	Duck	Partridge	Squab
Cornish hen	Goose	Pheasant	Turkey

Meat

Beef	Mutton	Pork	Venison

Mollusks

Abalone	Mussel	Scallop
Clam	Oyster	Squid

Shellfish

Crab	Crayfish	Lobster	Shrimp

Don't Be Caught By Cross-Contamination

When foods come into direct contact with each other, one food can end up with small amounts of allergenic substances from the other (the process is called "cross-contamination"). It takes only small amounts of some allergens to provoke a reaction, so even minor contact between foods can turn a "safe" food into an allergy trigger.

Cross-contamination can also make it difficult to identify food allergies correctly. If you react to a food that has not caused symptoms in the past, consider the possibility that the food has been contaminated by another one to which you actually are allergic.

The following examples describe some ways in which foods can become cross-contaminated:

- When several different foods are deep-fried in the same oil (as occurs often in restaurants), allergens from each food can be left behind in the oil and transferred to foods that are subsequently cooked in the oil. In this way, for example, french fries can be contaminated with egg proteins or fish proteins, resulting in an "unexplainable" allergic reaction. Whenever you order fried foods at a restaurant, always ask if other foods have been fried in the oil that will be used to cook your order. (Note: The cook may be the only one who knows the correct answer, so you may want to ask the cook yourself.)

- Countertops, cutting boards, dishes, serving utensils and food storage containers that have not been adequately washed between uses can retain foods on their surfaces. This problem occasionally causes people with food allergies to have allergic reactions in restaurants, where work surfaces and utensils are used many times with many different foods. To minimize this problem at home, it may be necessary to set up different work surfaces and provide different utensils and storage containers to ensure that an allergic member of the family is not exposed to the foods that trigger reactions. Care must also be taken during cooking, as steam and grease splatters can also cause cross-contamination.

- Food products stored together in the same container can cause cross-contamination. For example, this occurs easily if unwrapped cheeses, meats or baked goods are stored together in this way.

- In Chinese, Thai and Indian restaurants, there is a very high risk of cross-contamination due to the use of peanuts, tree nuts, fish and shellfish in a wide variety of dishes. If you are allergic to any of these foods, be extremely careful about eating in these ethnic restaurants.

- Cross-contamination can occur easily in restaurants where the same serving utensils are used to serve several different dishes — for example, when the same scoop is used to serve vanilla and peanut butter ice creams or the same salad spoon is used to serve tuna and chicken salads. Allergens can also be transferred when different serving utensils are allowed to come into contact with others, as occurs when different ice cream scoops are stored in the same bowl of water.

- Peanut allergies can be transferred from one candy to another if the trays that hold the candies or the machines that dispense them are not washed properly between candy changes.

When a Peanut is Your Worst Enemy

Peanuts are called an "exquisite allergen," because they need only be present in tiny quantities (as small as 1/44,000th of a peanut kernel) to cause severe reactions in people who are allergic to them (about one-third of peanut-sensitive people have these severe reactions). There are reports of peanut-sensitive people getting hives after contact with peanuts on unbroken skin, or having a reaction to airborne peanut protein in an airplane. Although some people outgrow allergies to other types of food (such as milk and wheat), an allergy to peanuts is usually lifelong.

Because it takes such small amounts of peanut protein to produce a strong reaction in some allergic people, if you are allergic to peanuts you must be aware of the numerous places where peanut allergens may crop up. Some examples:

- Peanut butter can be used as a thickener in such foods as chili, salsa, spaghetti sauce and gravies. It can also be found in egg rolls and prepackaged Rice Krispies® treats. (If you make these treats at home, use melted marshmallows instead of peanut butter to stick them together.)

- Peanut butter is sometimes used to give a crunchy texture to cheesecake crust, pie crust and some brands of brownies.

- Cross-contamination with peanuts can occur in equipment used to mix and manufacture chocolate products. Even if the machine is cleaned after peanuts are mixed in it, minute amounts of peanut may remain and get into the next batch of chocolate.

- Several different nut butters may be produced on the same production line. If peanut butter is made on the line, all subsequent nut butters could be cross-contaminated with peanut allergens. People who are allergic to peanuts should avoid all nut butters.

- Peanut oil is commonly used for cooking, especially in Chinese and Thai restaurants (where peanuts are also important ingredients in some dishes). Be aware that other foods cooked in the same oil, or even on the same grill, could expose you inadvertently to peanut allergen.

- Oils that are "cold-pressed" (a lower temperature process for extracting cooking oil) tend to have higher concentrations of nut protein. If you are allergic to peanuts, you should probably avoid this type of oil altogether.

What About Additives?

Today's processed foods contain thousands of additives. Some are put in to maintain freshness (since foods have to be transported greater distances); some are added to improve nutritional value (vitamins and minerals); others are included to make processing easier; and some are added simply to make foods look appealing.

These additives are considered safe for general consumption. Still, many people report reactions to some of these additives. Here are some of the additives commonly implicated in adverse reactions:

- Yellow dye No. 5 (tartrazine) used to color beverages, ice cream, desserts and other foods, has been reported to cause hives and swelling.

- Monosodium glutamate (MSG), used as a meat tenderizer and flavoring ingredient in Asian foods, has been alleged to trigger asthma episodes, but scientific studies have failed to confirm this. Such reactions to MSG may occur when people with asthma ingest it in combination with sulfites.

- Sulfites are used in some wines to control bacterial growth (and as preservatives to prevent food spoilage). Some people with asthma may have very strong reactions after ingesting sulfites, as sulfur dioxide is given off, causing reactions such as spasms of the bronchial tubes. Sulfites have also been associated, on rare occasions, with hives and anaphylaxis in patients with and without asthma.

- The artificial sweetner aspartame has been linked to allergic symptoms. However, carefully controlled studies have failed to show such an association. In a placebo-controlled clinical study involving volunteers who had previously reported aspartame-related symptoms, aspartame ingestion proved no more likely than placebo to cause hives. In another study, in which patients were given very high doses of aspartame, no clearly reproducible adverse reaction to aspartame could be identified. In short, in people who said they are allergic to aspartame, it's not clear if the symptoms are the result of allergic reaction or some other chemical reaction.

- BHT and BHA are antioxidants added to foods like breakfast cereals, and have been linked to allergic reactions in case reports. However, there is conflicting evidence of such associations. In a very small, placebo-controlled study, two patients with chronic hives were challenged with doses of BHT and BHA; exposures to these additives aggravated their symptoms, while withdrawal from them produced an abatement of the frequency and severity of their hives. However, a separate study found no convincing evidence of a link between BHT/BHA and allergies. As with aspartame, it's not clear if symptoms associated with BHT/BHA are the result of allergic reaction or some other chemical reaction.

START SLOWLY WITH YOUR BABY'S FOODS

If either or both parents have allergies, a baby's chances of developing them are increased. This risk can be reduced by withholding artificial formulas and solid food from your newborn until the age of six months, which gives the baby's immune system time to mature.

After six months, you can gradually begin to introduce solid foods by giving one new food at a time, waiting at least two to three days before starting the next one, according to the American Academy of Pediatrics (AAP). Watch for any possible adverse reactions, such as a new rash, respiratory problems, diarrhea, stomach upset or coughing, after a new food is tried. If these reactions occur, stop feeding the suspected food until you've talked with your pediatrician.

Here are some other suggestions from the AAP for introducing solid foods into your baby's diet. Begin with rice cereal (which is the least allergenic food), followed by oatmeal cereal and barley cereal. After that, a possible order is strained vegetables (start with squash, sweet potatoes and carrots), followed by fruit and then meat. Gradually, other foods can be added to the diet (although eggs are a good source of protein, initially feed your baby only the yolks, since they are not as likely to trigger allergies). Dairy products can become part of the diet at 12 months of age.

Food Allergies in Children

Will your baby develop allergies? As you've already read, food allergies occur in only a small minority of children—3 - 6% of those under age 3. Allergies, in fact, begin most frequently in the first and second years of life. One study found that allergies to cow's milk, eggs and fish start most often prior to the second year; allergies to fruits, vegetables and legumes tend to begin after the second year.

Allergic reactions to cow's milk or soy formula can appear within days to months after birth. In older children, a red, itchy, spotty rash may appear within 10-60 minutes of eating an allergenic food. Less common are respiratory symptoms associated with ingesting an allergen.

There is evidence that infants who are breastfed exclusively during the first 6 to 12 months of life develop less allergic disease by the age of 1 or 2 years than infants who are fed with formula. The American Academy of Pediatrics (AAP), in fact, recommends exclusive breastfeeding as ideal nutrition for about the first six months of life.

If you are nursing your baby, is it a good idea to avoid major allergenic foods, such as eggs and cow's milk? It depends on your baby. Some infants are so sensitive to certain foods that even the small amount that enters the mother's breast milk can cause a reaction (although this is rare). In these cases, mothers must avoid eating foods to which their babies are sensitive or allergic. According to the AAP, the best approach for the prevention of milk allergy in your infant is to breastfeed for as long as possible; milk allergies are rare among breast-fed babies.

If your baby develops allergic reactions to a formula, there are hypoallergenic formulas you can give your baby. Products like Nutramigen®

> # THE FOOD ALLERGY NETWORK
>
> The Food Allergy Network is a valuable resource for people with food aller-
> gies. This organization provides up-to-date reports on allergens in foods
> and food products in their newsletter, *The Food Allergy News*, and in *Special
> Food Allergy Alert!* notices. Contact the Network at: 10400 Eaton Place, Suite
> 107, Fairfax, VA 22030-2208, (800) 929-4040.

and Alimentum® are made for children and infants sensitive to cow's milk. Even though these formulas are considered safe, your physician may recommend giving them for the first time in his or her office, just in case there is an acute reaction.

Finally, keeping problem foods from your infant may not affect later development of certain respiratory conditions, such as allergic rhinitis or asthma. These are mostly due to inhaled allergens, as described in Chapter 2, and must be managed in a different way.

Keeping a Food Diary

Your doctor may ask you to keep a food diary as a tool to aid in diagnosing your food allergy, or as part of your treatment if you are starting an elimination diet. (Or, you may be keeping a diary for your child's daily food intake.) It is important to write down everything that you eat or drink so that important clues will not be missed. Make sure to write down all reactions; how soon after eating they occurred; and whether they are mild, moderate or severe. Rate your symptoms on a scale of 1 to 10. You may copy and use the form that follows, or devise your own. Since you will be using the diary several times each day, choose a size and format that will be portable and easy to use.

SAMPLE FOOD DIARY

Date
_____

Breakfast (time)
_____

Foods/Drinks consumed (and portions)
_____
_____
_____

Reactions (scale: 0 -10)/Timing (e.g., 1 hour after eating)
_____
_____
_____

Midmorning snack (time)
_____

Foods/Drinks consumed (and portions)
_____
_____
_____

Reactions (scale: 0 -10)/Timing (e.g., 1 hour after eating)
_____
_____
_____

Lunch (time)
_____

Foods/Drinks consumed (and portions)
_____
_____

Reactions (scale: 0 -10)/Timing (e.g., I hour after eating)

_____

_____

_____

Midafternoon snack (time)

_____

_____

Foods/Drinks consumed (and portions)

_____

_____

Reactions (scale: 0 -10)/Timing (e.g., I hour after eating)

_____

_____

_____

Dinner (time)

_____

_____

_____

Foods/Drinks consumed (and portions)

_____

_____

_____

Reactions (scale: 0 -10)/Timing (e.g., I hour after eating)

_____

_____

_____

After-dinner snack (time)

_____

_____

Foods/Drinks consumed (and portions)

_____

_____

_____

Reactions (scale: 0 -10)/Timing (e.g., 1 hour after eating)

_____

_____

_____

_____

Testing for Food Allergy

If you suspect you have a food allergy, it will take time to prove that it is a true allergy and to identify the specific problem food or foods. This is usually done through a process of testing and elimination of the suspected foods. The diagnostic process might look similar to the chart on the next page.

Other Treatments

Keep in mind that the best way of dealing with food allergies is to avoid the food(s) to which you're allergic. However, if you inadvertently consume an offending food, your doctor may recommend one or more medications that may relieve your symptoms. For example, if you develop hives (perhaps as part of a generalized allergic reaction that could also include a runny nose and other symptoms), you can take an over-the-counter antihistamine or consult your doctor. Cromolyn and corticosteroids are also sometimes recommended. Even so, these drugs are not always effective and they carry the risk of side effects. Thus, avoidance remains your best strategy.

DECISION TREE: FOLLOW THE REACTION

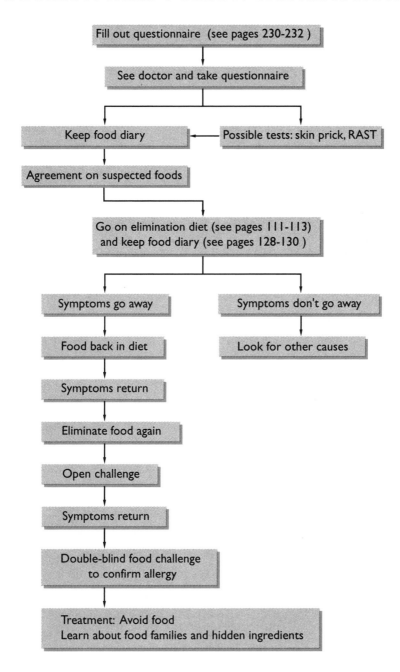

Chapter 7

Allergic Skin Reactions

Your skin is one of your body's most important organs, because it creates a physical barrier that protects you from damage by external agents such as bacteria, viruses and irritating or poisonous chemicals. But the protection your skin provides is not just physical in nature. Beneath the surface, your skin contains many immune cells — including mast cells. These cells provide additional protection against foreign "invaders" that get through the tough outer layer of skin.

Unfortunately, the immune cells within your skin can also work against you, if you are prone to allergies. Just as mast cells anywhere else in the body can react after exposure to an allergen, the mast cells in your skin can react and cause problems at any time you come in contact with the same allergen.

In fact, allergic skin reactions are extremely common (although the overwhelming majority of skin reactions are not due to allergy). Though usually not dangerous, allergic skin reactions can be extremely discomforting, resulting in itching, swelling, inflammation, rashes, hives, eczema and several other troublesome conditions. It's important to know when an allergy is responsible for a skin problem, because it can make a big difference in the way the problem is treated and may help you avoid future contact with the responsible allergen.

There are several different kinds of allergic skin reactions. The various reactions not only look different from one another, they also require different kinds of treatment. The most common allergic skin reactions include:

- Urticaria (hives)
- Angioedema
- Atopic dermatitis (eczema)
- Allergic contact dermatitis

Urticaria and Angioedema

Urticaria is the medical term used to describe the raised, red lesions that occur when an allergy or a physical event (such as exposure to cold) causes fluid (edema) to collect just beneath the surface of the skin. When the collection of fluid penetrates into the deep layers of the skin, causing more generalized swelling of an area, the condition is called angioedema.

Urticaria (Hives)

Urticaria is very common. It is estimated that 20 - 25% of the population have experienced an eruption of hives at some point during their lives. The lesions of urticaria (commonly known as "hives" or welts) can vary greatly in size and shape, but they almost always itch. Hives sometimes appear in clusters, and may have a "halo" or reddish area surrounding them. Typically, hives appear quickly after exposure to the offending allergen, and they usually leave quickly, too — within one to two hours. They rarely last over 24 hours. Some people may develop chronic urticaria, suffering repeated episodes over a long period of time (for example, six weeks or longer). When individual lesions persist longer than 24 hours, this can be a sign of another condition called urticarial vasculitis (explained later, in the section, *"Secondary" Hives*).

Angioedema

When the swelling (edema) that causes hives extends into the deeper layers of the skin, the condition is called angioedema. Most cases of angioedema cause only temporary swelling of the lips, eyes or face. In these locations, the swelling may be discomforting (and temporarily disfiguring), but is generally not dangerous. However, in rare cases, serious swelling can occur in the throat and airways, which can become life-threatening if it interferes with breathing. Angioedema usually lasts for a day or two, and hives may or may not be present at the same time.

Some rare cases of angioedema are hereditary. In these cases, the swelling may involve not only the tissues of the face and mouth, but also the respiratory and gastrointestinal tracts. When hereditary angioedema causes swelling of the skin, itching is not usually a problem, although the swelling may be painful. Intestinal swelling can cause nausea, vomiting, and severe abdominal cramping and pain.

The Causes of Hives and Angioedema

Hives and angioedema can be triggered by allergic reactions, physical irritants (such as physical pressure or exposure to heat or cold), psychological stress or by other medical conditions.

Allergic Triggers of Hives and Angioedema

When hives erupt shortly after a food or medication is ingested, the problem is almost always due to an allergic reaction. The most common allergic triggers of hives include:

- Foods such as peanuts and shellfish
- Insect bites and stings
- Medications, including a wide variety of over-the-counter drugs (aspirin and non-steroidal anti-inflammatory drugs are particularly frequent offenders), prescription drugs (most commonly, antibiotics) and even illicit drugs such as cocaine.

Physical Triggers of Hives and Angioedema

It is believed that the physical triggers of hives cause mast cells to release histamine in a different manner that does not involve the production of IgE antibodies. The most frequent triggers of hives include:

- Physical irritants, such as heat, cold, pressure, vibration, water and light
- Psychological factors, such as emotional stress
- Exercise

Physically-triggered hives have been divided into several different categories:

Dermatographism (skin writing) is a form of hives produced by stroking or rubbing of the skin, or even by simply scratching the skin or wearing tight-fitting clothes. In people with dermatographism, the skin will swell wherever pressure is applied. This form of urticaria affects about 5% of the population.

Cholinergic urticaria is triggered by increases in body temperature. Warm baths, hot tubs, exercise, emotions or fever can bring on hives in people with this condition. It is believed that raising the body temperature causes the increased release of acetylcholine, a chemical neurotransmitter that can stimulate mast cells. It starts as a small, measles-like rash, and scratching causes it to become hive-like. The rash may be accompanied by nausea, vomiting and diarrhea.

Cold-induced hives develop in some people after exposure to cold. Whatever part of the body is exposed can break out in hives. Simply drinking cold liquids can provoke swelling of the lips or mouth, either immediately or after a short period of time. This type of hives is sometimes accompanied by headache, low blood pressure, wheezing and nausea.

Solar hives occur after exposure to sunlight or a sunlamp. The lesions may erupt within a minute or two of the exposure.

Exercise-induced urticaria is a problem associated with physical activity. In some individuals a rash is the only sign of a problem. In others, a more serious condition called anaphylaxis may develop, with symptoms ranging from itching to breathing difficulties. In a few people, this problem will occur only if they have consumed a food to which they are allergic before they start exercising.

"Secondary" Hives

The appearance of hives (and many other rashes) can also be the consequence of another medical disorder. For this reason, a complete medical evaluation is appropriate whenever a simple explanation cannot be found for repeated episodes of urticaria or when hives are chronically persistent. Medical problems that can cause hives include the following:

- **Pruritic urticarial papules and plaques of pregnancy, or PUPP** is an itchy rash that occurs during the last trimester of pregnancy, typically starting over the central part of the abdomen and spreading to the buttocks and legs. This condition usually disappears shortly after delivery and does not usually recur with later pregnancies.

- **Idiopathic urticarial vasculitis** is a serious condition that causes tender hive-like welts on the hands, elbows, ankles and knees. These lesions may be accompanied by abdominal pain, nausea, vomiting, diarrhea, joint pain and stiffness. This problem is more prevalent in women than men.

- **Mastocytosis** is a systemic condition that results in the overproduction of mast cells by the body, which can cause hives.

If you break out in hives repeatedly, or they persist for more than 24 hours, you need to work with your doctor to identify the underlying cause. It is not always possible to identify what triggers hives, but your answers to the following questions will help your physician narrow the list of possibilities. Complete the following questionnaire and take it with you when you visit the doctor.

NOTE: If your skin breaks out on occasion and you are not sure whether the eruptions are hives, you should try to see your doctor while the lesions are still visible (or take a color picture of them). Even if you do not have an appointment, your doctor will probably be able to see you — even if just briefly — to confirm the diagnosis.

URTICARIA (HIVES) QUESTIONNAIRE

When was the first time you had hives?

_____

• Where were they located?

_____

•How many welts did you have?

_____

• Were you aware of anything that triggered the eruption?

_____

• How long did they last?

_____

• Did your doctor examine you, and what was the diagnosis?

_____

_____

• How were you treated?

_____

_____

Where do they typically appear on your body?

_____

_____

How long do the hives last?

_____

_____

How often do they recur?

_____

_____

_____

	Yes	No

Are you aware of anything that triggers your hives?

• Foods (If yes, list.)

• Medications (If yes, list.)

• Exercise

• Hot baths or hot tubs

• Exposure to cold

• Emotional stress

• Friction on your skin from tight-fitting clothes or rubbing

• Exposure to sunlight or a sunlamp

Have you taken any drugs, laxatives, vitamins or herbal products before the hives have appeared? (If yes, list.)

Does your skin appear normal after the hives go away?

What other problems do you notice when you have hives?

• Swelling of the eyes or face

• Swelling or itching of the lips, mouth, tongue or throat

• Difficulty swallowing

• Difficulty breathing

• Pain in the abdomen

• Nausea, vomiting or diarrhea

• Joint pain

The Treatment of Hives and Angioedema

The best way to deal with hives and angioedema is to identify and avoid the allergen or physical event that triggers the eruption. This can be simple when the outbreaks are far apart and occur only after you've eaten a particular food. When hives are persistent (lasting for six weeks or more) or recur very often, it may be impossible to identify the cause. However, you should see your doctor for a proper diagnosis and treatment guidance. Fortunately, chronic urticaria usually goes away by itself within six months, and most people are able to control the troublesome itching with simple self-care measures or medications.

Self-Care of Hives

Most people with occasional outbreaks of hives will get better on their own and require no treatment as long as they stay away from whatever triggered their outbreak. There are several measures you can use to relieve symptoms while the hives are subsiding (which rarely takes longer than 24 hours, and usually occurs much more rapidly):

- Wear loose, lightweight clothes.
- Try to work and sleep in a cool room.
- Take frequent showers or baths in lukewarm, not hot, water.
- Add colloidal oatmeal (brand name: Aveeno®) to the bath water for its soothing effect.
- Use gentle soaps (glycerine or cream) on your skin.
- Apply cooling creams or lotions to your skin immediately after you bathe, to trap moisture close to your skin.
- Avoid the use of aspirin and other non-steroidal anti-inflammatory drugs, such as ibuprofen — especially during outbreaks of hives. Between 20 - 40% of people with chronic urticaria are made worse by the use of these drugs.

Medical Treatment of Hives

When hives persist for long periods of time, or the symptoms (primarily itching) are very bothersome, the use of medications may be necessary for relief.

• The primary treatment for persistent or severely symptomatic hives involves the use of antihistamine drugs (see Chapter 5, pages 84-89). If you notice that your hives are most bothersome at a particular time of day (a common occurrence), talk with your doctor about the best time to take this medication, and how the timing of your symptoms may help in the diagnosis of the condition.

• When the symptoms of hives fail to respond to treatment with the commonly used nonsedating antihistamines, the following drugs may be useful:

— Doxepin: This tricyclic antidepressant medication is sometimes effective for treating chronic hives. However, unlike the commonly prescribed antihistamines that are nonsedating, this medication does tend to cause drowsiness.

— Hydroxyzine hydrochloride: This antianxiety agent has properties that may sometimes prove to be useful in treating chronic hives. But, like doxepin, it tends to cause drowsiness.

— Cyproheptadine: This sedating antihistamine has been shown to be useful in the treatment of cold-induced hives.

- If swelling of the mouth and throat accompanies an outbreak of hives, or angioedema interferes in any way with breathing, contact your doctor or go to the nearest emergency room immediately. The use of epinephrine (adrenaline) may be necessary to ensure that your airways are open sufficiently.

- Once an individual has experienced severe angioedema of the throat or airways, he or she should carry self-injectable epinephrine at all times (see Chapter 8, pages 172-174).

Atopic Dermatitis (Eczema)

Atopic dermatitis is a chronic skin disorder that affects infants and children more often than adults. According to the American Academy of Pediatrics, 10 - 12% of children between the ages of six months and 10 years are affected by eczema. Because the condition tends to improve with age, the estimated number of adults with eczema is only 0.7%. It is unusual for a person to develop eczema for the first time during adulthood.

Eczema is more common in people who have a family history of asthma or "hay fever" or who have these disorders themselves. An episode or eruption of eczema can be triggered by a number of different factors, including the following:

- Food allergies
- Environmental allergens such as dust mites, animal dander, molds or pollen
- Bacterial infections
- Heat or cold
- Stress

Several key signs and symptoms are characteristic of atopic dermatitis:
- Itching
- Dryness and scaling of the skin

- A typical pattern on the skin:

  — Infants: Widespread over the face, scalp, hands, arms and legs, and virtually over all of the body, but not the diaper area.
  — School-age children: In the creases of the elbows and knees; on the palms and soles, ankles, neck and face (especially the eyelids).
  — Adults: In the creases of the knees and elbows, on the neck, hands and feet.

- Over time, chronic inflammation and physical irritation (from scratching) can cause gradual thickening, scaling and darkening of the skin (ultimately, skin can develop a leathery texture).

- An increase in the incidence of skin infections (viral, fungal, bacterial).

- If the outer layer of the skin is damaged (as often happens because of excessive scratching), bacterial infections can easily develop, resulting in crusting and oozing.

Once atopic dermatitis appears in an area of the skin, a vicious cycle begins. Inflammation causes the already dry skin to lose more water, and makes the skin even drier. This weakens its ability to act as a barrier to allergens and irritants, so the damage increases. Several factors can aggravate atopic dermatitis:

- Low humidity, especially in the winter months
- High humidity, a special problem during the summer, because the skin reacts to the irritation of sweat
- Excessive body temperature
- Physical contact with wool or acrylic garments
- Physical contact with irritating chemicals
- Exposure to allergenic foods, airborne allergens and contact allergens
- Bacterial and viral infections in the eczematous lesions, especially by Staphylococcus aureus and Herpes simplex

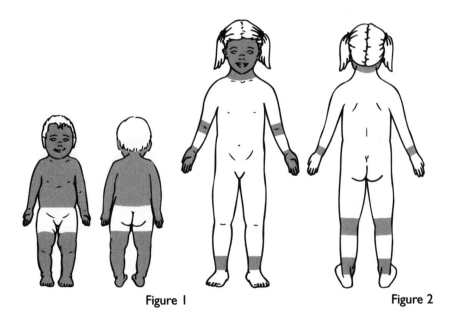

Figure 1   Figure 2

The areas of skin affected by atopic dermatitis tend to vary, depending on age. In infants, the dryness and scaling can be widespread over the body, although it usually is not present in the diaper area (see Figure 1). School-age children with eczema are most likely to have lesions in the creases of the elbows and knees, and on the palms and soles, the ankles, and the neck and face (see Figure 2).

- Emotional stress
- Scratching, which perpetuates the itching it is intended to relieve, and — in the process — damages the underlying skin and produces inflammation

Diagnosing Eczema

There is no single test that can diagnose eczema with complete accuracy. However, the diagnosis can usually be made based on a complete

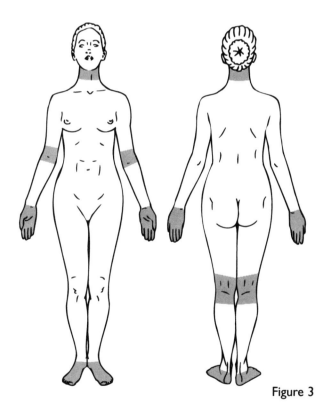

Figure 3

In adults, atopic dermatitis appears most commonly on the neck, hands and feet, and in the creases of the elbows and knees (see Figure 3).

medical history and thorough physical exam (see Chapter 4). If questions remain, the following tests and procedures may provide additional evidence:

- Blood tests for IgE may reveal elevated levels (80% of people with atopic dermatitis have abnormally high levels of IgE).

- Skin prick tests can be performed for suspected allergens. This approach is only practical when the list of suspected allergens has been narrowed down to a reasonable number. Skin tests on people with atopic dermatitis must be interpreted with caution as they have a high percentage of false positive results. The test may erroneously demonstrate an allergy to a particular substance when one does not exist.

- Radioallergosorbent (RAST) blood tests can be performed for suspected allergens. These tests must also be interpreted with caution because of the high false positive rate in people with eczema (due to high IgE levels).

- Elimination diets can be used when food allergens are suspected of provoking the eczema. In some patients, the skin lesions will improve when the offending allergen is removed from the diet. Elimination diets are much more likely to produce results in children than adults, because food allergy resulting in eczema is more common in children.

- Dust mite control can be exerted, and may improve the condition (mites are a known allergic factor in this disorder).

Self-Care of Eczema (Atopic Dermatitis)

In the majority of people with eczema, the skin disorder gradually disappears over a period that can range from a few months to a few years. The healing process is likely to move more quickly if the underlying trigger for the eczema—such as a food allergen—can be identified and eliminated. But even if that cannot be done, there are many ways to relieve the symptoms while the process resolves itself. Here are several things you can do on your own to obtain relief:

- Moisturize your skin by bathing or showering at least once a day in lukewarm water (hot water increases skin dryness); bear in mind, however, that some people do better with less bathing.

- Avoid the use of bubble baths and harsh soaps which can aggravate dry skin; look for pH-neutral soaps instead.

- After a bath or shower, pat your skin dry (do not rub) and apply an emollient cream or ointment (such as mineral oil or white petrolatum) to help the skin retain moisture.

- Avoid sunburn or excessive exposure to artificial ultraviolet light.

- Use air conditioning in your home during the summer and humidify the air during the winter.

- Reduce your exposure to airborne allergens such as pollens, molds, dust mites, cockroaches and animal dander.

- Try to reduce your stress levels. Stress can exacerbate symptoms in some cases. Obtain professional counseling if necessary.

- Keep your fingernails short to minimize the damage that occurs when you scratch the affected areas, almost automatically, while sleeping. For children, some pediatricians recommend placing cotton socks over the hands at bedtime.

- Contact your doctor immediately if any areas of skin become infected, or if areas of eczema become crusted, "weepy" or oozy. Your doctor may recommend the use of compresses soaked in Burow's solution or cool saline solution to loosen the crusts and soften the skin.

- Do not use any ointment or cream to treat areas of atopic dermatitis without talking to your doctor first. Many products that are commonly used to treat skin infections or inflammation (and commonly found in medicine cabinets) can actually make atopic dermatitis worse by creating an allergic contact dermatitis on top of the existing problem (see next section). These products include topical antibiotics such as neomycin and bacitracin; topical anesthetics such as benzocaines; and topical antihistamines such as diphenhydramine. In addition, fragrances and preservatives in these products and in simple moisturizers and cosmetic creams can produce allergic reactions.

- Check with your doctor before applying anything to an area of skin affected by eczema. The skin of some areas of the body, especially the face, armpits and groin, can be permanently injured by ointments or creams containing strong steroid preparations. Consult with your doctor before applying a steroid preparation to these areas.

Medical Treatment of Atopic Dermatitis

If self-care measures fail to provide adequate relief within a reasonable amount of time (2-3 weeks) or if the eczema is severe, your physician may recommend that treatment with medications be initiated.
The options available include the following:

- Topical (applied directly to the skin) corticosteroids are considered the primary treatment for atopic dermatitis. Many different
  creams, lotions and ointments are available in a wide variety of
  strengths. Your doctor will help you select one that is most
  appropriate for your particular problem. Typically, high-potency
  steroids are used on the skin for about a week, followed by up to
  2 to 3 weeks of treatment with a milder dose. Topical steroids
  need to be applied cautiously to the face and genitals and over
  skin-fold areas. In children, low-potency products are preferred,
  and caution must be used if the eczema covers large areas of an
  infant's skin, or an area that would be covered by a diaper.

- If necessary, your doctor may also recommend or prescribe an
  oral medication to help relieve the itching.

In people who have eczema that fails to improve with the measures
described above, a trial of phototherapy may be considered. This
involves medically-supervised ultraviolet light exposure, sometimes in
combination with orally-taken psoralens (chemical substances that
enhance the effects of the ultraviolet rays). Phototherapy is generally used only to treat severe cases of eczema that do not respond to
simpler treatments because the ultraviolet radiation can produce pre-
mature wrinkling of the skin, freckling and an increased risk of skin
cancer.

Contact Dermatitis: Allergy or Irritant?

The medical term "dermatitis" means simply "inflammation of the skin." It is used by doctors to describe a complex set of microscopic cellular and chemical reactions that occur when tissues in the body are injured. But in ordinary terms, inflammation refers to the redness, swelling and pain you can observe after an injury or infection. You have probably seen inflammation many times yourself. Inflammation is what causes the redness after a burn, the swelling and pain of a boil and the redness of a sore throat. With regard to contact dermatitis, inflammation is seen as a "rash."

There are many different causes of dermatitis, but this book will cover only two: *irritant contact dermatitis* and *allergic contact dermatitis,* both of which involve skin inflammation that follows direct contact with a foreign substance. The two conditions may actually look quite similar, but there are some significant differences between them:

- **In irritant contact dermatitis,** the inflammation results from a direct physical injury to the skin by an irritating or toxic substance (an example would be the inflammation that follows direct contact with a strong acid or lye). Irritant contact dermatitis occurs very frequently, because it can be caused by a wide variety of natural and man-made substances. The most common causes of this form of dermatitis are solvents, and exposure often occurs in the workplace. But many of the products used at home can produce the same results; "dish-pan hands," for example, is a reaction to the irritants in detergents.

COMMON CAUSES OF ALLERGIC CONTACT DERMATITIS

Plants

- Plants from the Toxicodendron genus: Poison ivy, poison oak, poison sumac

Rubber and Rubber Products

- Mercaptobenzothiazole
- Carbamates
- Thiurams
- Black rubber paraphenylene diamine

Medications

- Antibiotic creams and ointments (neomycin, bacitracin)
- Anesthetic creams and ointments (benzocaine)
- Corticosteroid creams and ointments
- Thimerosal
- Quinolines

Cosmetics

- Fragrances (Cinnamic aldehyde, Balsam of Peru)
- Cosmetic bases and carrier vehicles (preservatives, lanolin, imidazolidinyl urea, formaldehyde, parabens, quaternium-15, ethylenediamine dihydrochloride)
- Hair dyes (p-phenylenediamine)

Metals

- Nickel
- Potassium dichromate
- Cobalt

Resins

- Colophony
- p-tert-butylphenol formaldehyde resin
- Epoxy resin

- **In allergic contact dermatitis,** the inflammation occurs because you have been previously sensitized to the substance and the current contact triggers an immune response (an example might be the swelling and redness that would occur around your eyes if you kept using mascara to which you had become allergic; when you touch poison ivy, the subsequent redness and itching is another example of this skin allergy). Allergic contact dermatitis is less common than the irritant form, but there are still nearly 3,000 chemicals that can produce an immune response leading to this problem.

Irritant or Allergic: How to Tell the Difference

The rashes caused by physical irritation and allergic reactions are often similar in appearance: both have redness, swelling and blisters. A complete medical history and thorough physical examination may help your doctor determine which type of reaction is producing the rash.

In some cases, the history and physical alone will identify the cause of a rash. (For example, a circular-shaped rash on your wrist directly under your stainless steel watch is a clear sign that you are allergic to nickel in the watch casing.) In other instances, the diagnosis will not be so clear. That's when skin testing can help determine if an allergy exists.

The skin tests are done by applying patches containing suspected allergens directly to the skin for 24-96 hours, and observing to see which — if any — produce an inflammatory reaction. Since it is not possible to test for every one of the 3,000 substances known to produce allergic contact dermatitis, your doctor will need to identify the most likely allergen suspects. Your medical history and physical examination will help the doctor narrow the list.

Before visiting the doctor, gather the information from the following questionnaire and bring it with you to your visit:

CONTACT DERMATITIS QUESTIONNAIRE

Family History

• Do either or both of your parents have allergies?

One Parent_____   Both Parents_____   Neither Parent_____

Past History

	Yes	No
• Have you had any kind of allergic reaction in the past?		
• Have you experienced the same kind of rash in the past?		

• If so, when did it occur, how long did it last, what was the diagnosis, and how many times has it recurred?

_____

_____

_____

Occupational Exposures

	Yes	No
• Does your work expose you to physical contact with any chemicals, solvents or resins?		
• Did your rash occur after the use of a new chemical or solvent at work?		
• Did the rash occur after an accidental exposure to a chemical or solvent (for example, after tearing a hole in a protective glove)?		

	Yes	No

Household Exposures

• Do you have any new carpets or furniture that might
contain formaldehyde or other irritants or allergens?

• Have you done any repairs around the house that involved the use
of glues, solvents, paints or paint thinners?

• Have you used any acids or lye to clean objects or clear drains?

• Have you used any new or different household cleaning agents,
such as detergents, metal cleaners or soaps?

Hobby Exposures

• Do you use glues, solvents, dyes or paints to make handicrafts?

• Have you used any new or different products in your hobbies?

Clothing and Jewelry

• Have you noticed a rash after wearing certain clothes or jewelry?

• Did your rash appear after purchasing a new article
of clothing or jewelry?

Cosmetics

• Do you break out on occasions when you use makeup?

• Have you switched brands of cosmetics, or purchased
new items that you have not used previously?

• Does your rash disappear if you stop using makeup
for periods of time?

Yes   No

Outdoor Exposures

• Do you work in the garden with plants that can cause
  irritant or allergic reactions?

• Do you use chemicals and fertilizers in your gardening?

• Is there a pattern between your work in the garden
  or your use of chemicals there and the outbreak of a rash?

• Did you obtain any plants or use any new chemicals prior
  to the appearance of your rash?

• Do you frequently go camping or hiking?

• Did your rash follow a hike into the brush or a camping trip?

Topical Products or Medications

• Did your rash appear after the use of a topical medication
  (cream, lotion or ointment)?

• Have you used any antibiotic or anesthetic creams?

• Are you using any over-the-counter creams or lotions
  (including moisturizers, sunscreens, medicated shampoos)?

• Did the rash occur in an area where you have previously used
  topical products or medications?

Physical Signs

• **Timing of the rash:** Did the inflammation appear soon
  after contact with a particular substance?

When dermatitis is the result of direct irritation, especially when extremely
irritating or corrosive substances are involved, the inflammation appears

shortly after contact with the substance. When allergy is responsible, the appearance of inflammation is usually delayed. (For example, the allergic skin reaction to poison oak or poison ivy usually begins about 24-48 hours after the exposure, but it can appear as late as 7-10 days later.)

• **Distribution of the rash:** Shade the areas of the body where the rash appears. Identifying where the rash appears may provide some of the best clues about the specific cause of the inflammation.

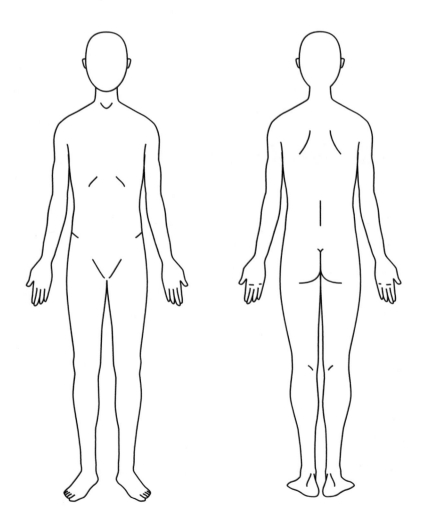

OTHER SKIN PROBLEMS THAT MIMIC ALLERGIC CONTACT DERMATITIS

Several other skin conditions can mimic the signs and symptoms of allergic contact dermatitis. These include:

- **Seborrheic dermatitis:** Usually associated with oily skin, it appears on the scalp and around the nose (in infants, it may occur on the neck and diaper area).
- **Atopic dermatitis:** See pages 142-149 in this chapter.
- **Photosensitive dermatitis:** Skin eruptions that result from interactions between chemicals or drugs and ultraviolet light. Common triggers include sulfa drugs, tetracycline, coal tar extract and psoralens. The rash resembles eczema, with drying, scaling and peeling.

- Most cases of irritant contact dermatitis involve the skin on the hands, since the hands are usually the first part of the body to come into contact with irritants. Allergic reactions often involve the face, hands and feet.

- Allergic reactions to nickel typically appear in areas that are in contact with metal jewelry containing nickel (watches, earrings, necklaces). The common areas affected are the wrists, neck and earlobes. Nickel allergy can also cause inflammation under the breasts in women who wear underwire bras.

- Allergic reactions to medications usually involve areas where the offending cream, lotion or ointment has been applied. If you did not wash your hands after applying the medication, a rash may also appear at any other location you touched afterward (the face, especially around the eyes, is a common area affected).

- A band-like rash around the waist is usually due to an allergic reaction to formaldehyde in the elastic waistband of underwear.

- A rash on the top of the foot is often due to contact with potassium dichromate, a chemical used to tan leather for shoes.

The Treatment of Contact Dermatitis

Whatever the cause of contact dermatitis — irritant or allergy — the first step in managing the problem is to remove the offending substance and prevent all further contact with it. In the case of an allergen like poison ivy, this means not only staying away from the plant itself, but washing the toxic oil off any other objects that came in contact with the plant (like the clothing you wore and the dog who walked through the brush with you).

The treatment of the rash itself is focused on reducing the inflammation and providing symptomatic relief. Topical corticosteroid creams are the first choice to combat the inflammation. They are available in various potencies, and your doctor can determine the appropriate choice for treating your condition.

If an allergic contact rash is very extensive or it involves the face or genital area, systemic corticosteroid drugs (taken orally) will need to be used. Typically, these medications are prescribed for 5 to 10 days, starting with a higher dose that gradually tapers downward. Your doctor should be your guide on any medication you use for allergic contact dermatitis.

For symptomatic relief, cool, moist compresses can be applied directly to the area of the rash. A soft, clean cloth (such as a handkerchief) should be soaked in cool water. This should be repeated 2-4 times a day for 10-15 minutes at a time. After compressing the area, it should be gently patted dry (not rubbed), and the steroid cream applied. Once the inflammation diminishes (which can take 3-4 days), the compresses can be discontinued and the steroid cream used alone. It may take two weeks for the rash to clear completely, although associated symptoms, such as itching, may subside more rapidly.

Oral antihistamines may help relieve the itching in allergic contact dermatitis. Topical antihistamine and antibiotic creams should not be applied to an area of contact dermatitis, as this can actually aggravate the already inflamed skin.

Poison Ivy, Oak and Sumac

Perhaps the best-known cause of allergic contact dermatitis is the toxicodendron group of plants, which includes poison ivy, poison oak, eastern poison oak and poison sumac. Notable for their three-leaf clusters, these plants contain an oily resin called urushiol, which is responsible in sensitized people for the blisters and itchy, red rash that appear after contact with the plants. The resin penetrates the skin (even in the absence of cuts) and combines with proteins, setting the process of sensitization into motion. White blood cells gather where the allergen first entered and then travel to other parts of your body. These are the cells that are activated and produce an allergic reaction when you have future contact with poison ivy, poison oak or sumac.

Interestingly, minor contact with the plants is not enough to trigger the allergic reaction in many people. In fact, it takes more than one exposure before most people will develop a rash. But most people will develop a rash after a major exposure to urushiol, or after repeat-

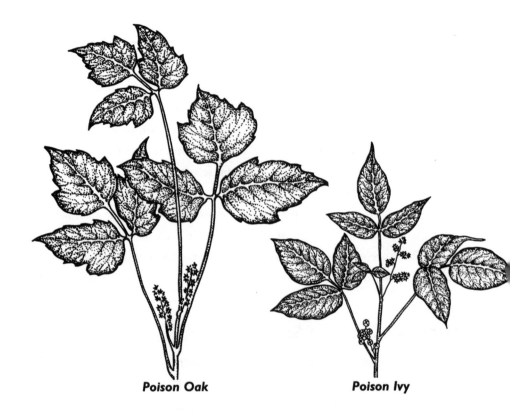

Poison Oak   **Poison Ivy**

ed minor exposures to the resin. If a reaction does occur after only one contact, it takes 7-10 days before the rash develops. Once a person has been sensitized, the rash will occur within 48 hours after another exposure.

"Leaves of three, let them be," is the familiar chant of campers, but you don't have to come in direct contact with the plant itself to develop allergic contact dermatitis. The resin can also adhere to your clothing if you brush up against the plants, or to the fur of pets if they make contact. If you're not careful when removing your clothing, or you pet the animal before washing the resin off its coat, a rash can develop that is just as troublesome as if your skin had made direct contact with the plant itself.

Rashes that are caused by contact with urushiol are much more common during the spring, summer and fall, because these are the times when toxicodendron plants are growing, their leaves are plentiful, and people are most likely to come in contact with them. However, the risk is also present during the winter, because active resin remains in dead and dormant plants.

If resin becomes trapped under your fingernails, scratching healthy skin around the rash or elsewhere will create new lesions. However, if you scratch the blisters in a poison ivy rash, this will not spread the eruption from one part of the body to another or to another person, as the blisters do not contain any of the toxic resin. (Taking injections of the plant, immunotherapy, doesn't prevent a reaction due to urushiol contact.)

Self-Care of Rashes Due to Urushiol Contact

The allergic rash caused by exposure to urushiol typically reaches its peak within five days, and symptoms are likely to be worse at this time. If left alone, the rash will usually heal by itself within two weeks. There are several things you can do to minimize the severity of the rash, decrease the risk of spreading the lesions, relieve symptoms and speed the healing process:

- The first thing to do after contact with any of the plants containing urushiol is to eliminate the resin from your clothes (including gloves and shoes) and your skin. If you wash the resin from your skin within five minutes, it is highly unlikely that you will develop a rash. Even if you can't wash it off that quickly, do so at the first opportunity, as this will minimize the risk of spreading resin to other parts of the body.

- Carefully remove and wash all clothes that have come in contact with the resin, including gloves and shoes. Wash any other garments that may have come in contact with the clothes that touched the plants. (Urushiol can be transferred from one garment to another—for example, when packing them together in a suitcase or backpack.)

- Wash all camping gear that may have come in contact with urushiol or the toxicodendron group of plants. The resin can remain active and allergenic for up to a year.

- Use cold, wet compresses to relieve symptoms and reduce inflammation. (You cannot spread the rash this way.)

- Apply calamine lotion to help control itching.

Medical Treatment of Rashes
Due to Urushiol Contact

If the rash is on your face or genital area, or if the rash covers more than 20% of your body, consult your physician. Your physician may recommend the use of topical corticosteroids. Or, if the rash is severe or extensive, your physician may prescribe treatment with systemic steroids (taken orally).

Preventing Contact with Urushiol

Despite the well-known hazards of skin contact with urushiol, rashes caused by toxicodendron plants are extremely common.

Here are some simple tips for preventing contact:

- Become familiar with the appearance of plants in the genus toxicodendron so that you have no difficulty recognizing and avoiding them in the future.

- Do not gather kindling or firewood near poison oak, ivy or sumac plants. Resin transferred from the plants will be vaporized and can contact your skin where exposed, resulting in the typical rash.

- If you are allergic to urushiol, be aware that you may also react to other plants in the same family of trees (the cashew family). These include cashew, mango and Japanese lacquer trees. Sensitive people may react after peeling mangoes, or after handling lacquered wood products from Japan or China.

- If you are sensitive to urushiol, do not personally clear your yard or grounds of poison oak, ivy or sumac plants; have someone else do it. Be especially careful when clearing ground during the winter, as these plants are dormant and have no recognizable leaves.

- Do not rely on over-the-counter lotions and creams that are sold as protective "barriers" against urushiol. These products do not offer 100% protection, and they can be rendered less effective by perspiration or abrasion.

Latex: The "New" Allergy

Latex, the milky white sap from the Brazilian rubber tree, is a major ingredient in rubber products. Latex is present almost everywhere in the modern environment — including condoms, surgical gloves,

COMMON LATEX PRODUCTS
AT HOME AND WORK

Latex is difficult to avoid today, because it is present in a very broad range of products. The following list includes some commonly used products that contain natural rubber latex. If you are allergic to latex, you should do everything possible to avoid further contact with any object that contains it. In almost all cases, alternative products are available that are not made with latex (for example, garments containing synthetic elastic fibers such as spandex and natural skin condoms).

Adhesive bandages and tape

Baby bottle nipples

Balloons

Carpet and rug backing

Condoms

Diaper fasteners
 (disposable diapers)

Diaphragms

Douche bulbs

Elastic in clothing

Erasers

Eyedropper bulbs

Hot water bottles

Koosh® balls

Pacifiers

Paints

Rubber bands

Rubber clothing
 (such as raincoats, galoshes)

Rubber gloves

Rubber toys

Rubber handgrips on racquets, bicycles, garden tools, shop tools and other objects

Shoes made with rubber

adhesive bandages, rubber bands, shoes and balloons. And latex allergy is on the rise — in large part because of the increasing use of latex by healthcare workers.

The symptoms of latex allergy may be immediate, occurring within minutes of the contact, or delayed for up to 12 hours. The severity of the symptoms and signs of latex allergy depend on the amount of latex allergen entering the body. Symptoms may include:

- Hives or itchy welts
- Stuffy, runny nose, sneezing and itching of the nose, eyes or roof of the mouth
- Wheezing, coughing and shortness of breath
- Anaphylaxis and shock

If you are allergic to latex, you should carefully avoid any further exposure to this substance, especially if previous reactions have resulted in difficulty breathing, low blood pressure or anaphylaxis. The following steps will help you prevent further exposure to latex:

- Notify all healthcare professionals in writing of your allergy to latex. Be sure to include not only your primary care physician, but all specialists, dentists and allied health professionals whom you see on a regular basis. Be sure to tell all new physicians about your latex allergy, and remind every doctor about it each time you have an appointment, including physicians you are seeing only for diagnostic tests (such as radiologists). Many of the instruments used in diagnostic testing may contain some latex.

- Notify your pharmacist in writing of your allergy to latex and request that this information be added to your "patient profile."

(Most pharmacies keep a computerized profile on all customers that includes information about allergies.)

- If you have a medical chart at a local community hospital, notify the hospital in writing of your allergy to latex and request that this information be added to your chart.

- Purchase and carry vinyl gloves with you to all medical and dental appointments, in case your doctor or dentist only has latex gloves available in the office. (Request that vinyl gloves be made available at subsequent visits.)

- Wear a Medic Alert bracelet or pendant that indicates you are allergic to latex. (This can be lifesaving in the event you are unconscious and require emergency medical treatment.)

- If you have experienced an anaphylactic reaction after exposure to latex, talk to your doctor about the possible need to carry an automatic epinephrine injector at all times (see pages 172-174 for a more complete discussion of this subject).

Chapter 8

Insect Bites & Stings and Anaphylaxis

Few people get through life without being stung by an insect, and most of us are stung more than once. Although everyone who is stung has to endure some amount of pain and discomfort, people who are allergic to insect venom can suffer serious (and in some cases life-threatening) complications. Experts think that about 3% of adults and 1% of children are at risk of suffering serious allergies to insect stings and attribute about 50 deaths every year in the United States to severe allergic reactions caused by stings.

Allergic reactions to insect stings do not occur the first time you are stung. These reactions develop only after the immune system has become sensitized to the insect's venom, and this requires your having been stung before. Even if the only sting you have suffered was years ago, you could still experience an allergic reaction if you are stung again.

The Insects

Stinging insects can be broadly divided into two different categories: vespids and apids. Vespids include the yellow jacket, the hornet and the wasp, while apids include the honeybee and the bumblebee. Any of these insects can trigger allergic reactions in certain people. Some people are allergic to all of them, others to only one or two. Of all stinging insects the yellow jacket is the most common cause of allergic reactions. Yellow jackets nest in the ground and are easily disturbed in the course of routine activities like gardening.

Biting insects, like mosquitoes, rarely cause serious allergic reactions.

Fire ants can cause severe allergic reactions and are increasing in numbers in the United States, particularly in the southeast. Fire ants both bite and sting. They first attach themselves to the skin by biting, then sting their victim multiple times.

Reactions to Insect Stings

Normal reactions: Typically, insect stings cause mild redness, pain or swelling at the site of the sting. The reaction is usually brief and generally subsides within several hours.

The normal reaction to fire ants is quite characteristic. Immediately following a sting, a small hive forms which then develops into a fluid-filled blister that gradually dries up over a period of several days.

Large local reactions: In some people, insect stings can cause extensive swelling and redness over a large area around the site of the sting. The symptoms may gradually worsen for the first day or two after the sting and can last as long as a week to ten days. Some people who develop very severe local reactions may also experience nausea and fatigue.

Anaphylaxis: Insect stings can cause a potentially life-threatening anaphylactic reaction. Symptoms of anaphylaxis caused by insect stings vary from person to person. The most common symptoms involve only the skin and include hives, flushing and swelling. However, more serious symptoms affecting the respiratory and cardiovascular systems can occur, leading to a dangerous drop in blood pressure and difficulty breathing. Symptoms of anaphylaxis usually occur within 15 minutes of the sting and, if not treated quickly, can be deadly (see pages 172-174 for more about anaphylaxis).

Diagnosing an Insect Sting Allergy

The diagnosis of an insect sting allergy can usually be made based on your history of previous sting reactions. Your physician will want to know the timing of your stings, the types of symptoms you experienced as a result of the stings, and what occurs during the course of the reaction. Even so, he or she may have difficulty identifying the exact culprit.

When an insect sting allergy is suspected, skin testing should be performed to confirm the diagnosis and guide proper treatment. Skin testing involves placing a small amount of the insect venom under the skin and monitoring your body's response to it. Special venom extracts of honeybee, yellow jacket, yellow hornet, baldface hornet and wasp are available for this type of testing. A fire ant extract is also available for people with suspected fire ant allergies. Since people who are allergic to one type of insect are often allergic to others as well, and the insects are difficult to tell apart, testing should always be performed by a doctor using each of the different venoms.

Treating an Insect Sting Allergy

Avoidance: When an insect allergy is diagnosed, the most important thing is to avoid being stung again. Simple precautions can go a long way in preventing a re-sting. For example, covering up as much as possible when you are outdoors puts a physical barrier between you and the insects. Wear long pants, shirts with long sleeves and shoes when you are outdoors. Avoid yellow or black clothing, and do not walk barefoot. Use gloves when you garden. Do not wear perfume. And be extremely careful whenever you decide to cook or eat outside — the smell of food is sure to attract insects.

Medical therapy: A normal mild reaction to a sting can be treated simply by applying cold compresses to the affected area and using over-the-counter analgesics (such as aspirin or ibuprofen) to help alleviate discomfort and control swelling. Some doctors also recommend the use of antihistamines. Large local reactions are treated similarly. However, steroid medications may be indicated if the reaction is particularly severe.

In the case of anaphylactic reactions, a medication called epinephrine must be administered as quickly as possible after the symptoms of anaphylaxis appear, and medical attention should be sought. People who have suffered anaphylactic reactions to stings should carry epinephrine with them and be prepared to self-administer the medication if they are stung, even before symptoms appear. People experiencing their first anaphylactic reaction should seek out emergency medical care immediately.

Venom immunotherapy: A procedure called venom immunotherapy has been shown to be highly effective in preventing repeat anaphylactic reactions to stinging insects and fire ants. It involves actually giving an allergic person the venom which he or she is allergic to. Initially, very small doses of the venom are given. The doses are then increased until a maintenance dose is reached.

Immunotherapy should include each venom to which an individual is sensitive as determined by skin testing. Although your allergy specialist will determine the appropriate length of treatment for you, therapy should generally be continued (with maintenance doses given every four weeks during the first year of therapy, every six weeks during the second year and every eight weeks after that) until the skin test becomes negative or after three to five years. If the maintenance shots are stopped earlier, protection against an anaphylactic reaction is often lost.

YOUR CHILD & INSECT STINGS

Children who are stung by a bee, wasp or yellow jacket have less of a tendency to develop a life-threatening anaphylactic reaction than adults. After an individual experiences a first sting, the insect venom sensitizes him or her, setting the stage for an allergic reaction if a subsequent sting occurs; however, the chances of having a severe reaction with a second sting are less in children than in adults. For that reason, when deciding whether venom immunotherapy is appropriate for a particular patient, many doctors use more stringent criteria with children.

Keep in mind, however, that serious reactions can occur in children, so precautions such as keeping epinephrine kits at hand make sense if your child is allergy-prone.

Immunotherapy is not without risks. A small number of people develop anaphylactic reactions to the very small doses given at the beginning of treatment; others develop anaphylaxis as the doses of venom are increased. A more common reaction is uncomfortable, local swelling and redness. Following a severe reaction to treatment, the next dose is reduced significantly and subsequent doses are increased more gradually. In rare cases, the treatment must be stopped entirely.

Anaphylaxis

The symptoms of anaphylaxis may vary in their severity, but the reaction is usually dramatic and immediate. As massive amounts of histamine are released within the body, the person may first experience tingling or itching in the mouth, followed quickly by more serious symptoms such as vomiting and diarrhea. Blood vessels throughout the body dilate, causing blood pressure to fall quickly. Swelling of the throat and airways occurs frequently, obstructing breathing and contributing to a major medical emergency. Wheezing, coughing, and swelling of the legs, hands, feet and eyes may also occur. If appropriate action is not implemented immediately, death can occur.

The most important immediate step is the injection of epinephrine, which is an antidote to the histamine. Several automatic epinephrine injectors are available for self-administration, and you should be prepared to administer this medication yourself at the first sign of an anaphylactic episode. Expert help should be summoned immediately, also, either from others in the immediate area or by calling 911.

After self-injecting epinephrine, an immediate visit to the nearest emergency room is imperative, because the drug will wear off in a short time and other medical treatment may be necessary.

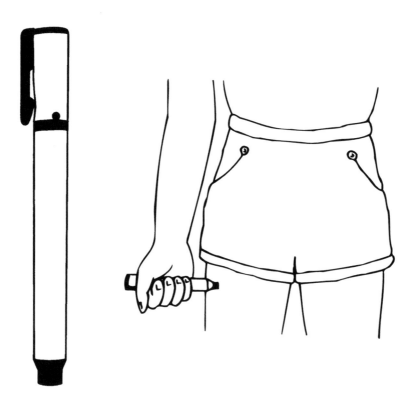

The *Epi-E•Z Pen®* is a semi-automatic device that can be used to self-inject epinephrine. The built-in syringe contains a pre-measured dose of epinephrine, which is rapidly injected into the body when the spring mechanism is set and the device is firmly pressed against a leg muscle (the medication can even be injected through clothing, if necessary). A training device, which comes without a needle or medication, is available for practice.

Epinephrine injectors are available only by prescription. They should be used only for emergency supportive care (for example, to treat anaphylactic reactions that interfere with breathing or cause blood pressure to fall). Your physician will provide you with guidelines for when and how this device should be used. Use of the device does not eliminate the need for immediate follow-up medical care.

Once you have experienced an anaphylactic reaction, you should always carry an injectable form of epinephrine with you. Most life-threatening anaphylactic reactions occur away from home. For this reason, you should keep two epinephrine kits with you at all times, in a jacket pocket or in your purse. (You may have to repeat the treatment 20 minutes after the first one.)

Your physician can prescribe the prefilled epinephrine injector systems (EpiPen®, Epi-E•Z Pen® or Ana-Kit®). You should purchase extra kits and keep them in key locations, such as your desk at work and the glove compartment of your car. Inspect your kits on a regular basis, and replace them as soon as the expiration date is reached. (If the kit has become discolored, discard it and replace it even if the expiration date has not been reached.)

Your doctor or pharmacist should teach you how to use the kit. Then you should teach family members and your closest coworkers and friends how to use it — just in case you are not able to do it yourself during an anaphylactic reaction.

If your child is allergic, keep epinephrine kits (EpiPen Jr.® 0.15 mg) at school and at the baby-sitter's house. Make sure that school personnel and the baby-sitter know how to respond to an anaphylactic reaction, including the administration of the epinephrine.

Anyone who has had an anaphylactic reaction should also wear a Medic Alert bracelet or pendant. This simple device can make the difference between life and death if you are unconscious when medical help arrives. For more information, call Medic Alert at 1-800-633-4260.

Chapter 9

Drug Allergies

Adverse drug reactions are exceptionally common. Up to 30% of people taking medications experience some sort of adverse reaction. However, less than 10% of these are due to true drug allergies involving the immune system. The remainder have other causes that need to be managed differently (see box on page 176).

Contrary to popular belief, allergic drug reactions do not occur the first time you take a medication. Allergies develop only after the immune system has had a chance to respond to the drug by producing specific IgE antibodies against it. Once these drug-specific antibodies attach themselves to mast cells—a process that can occur within hours—you are "sensitized" to the drug, and any further exposure to that same drug will trigger an allergic reaction.

Signs and Symptoms of a Drug Allergy

Drug allergies can cause a wide variety of symptoms and signs. Symptoms are something you feel or experience subjectively, like itching or nausea, but they cannot be seen. Signs are objective changes that can be seen, such as a rash or swelling.

ADVERSE DRUG REACTIONS

Predictable Adverse Drug Reactions

Side effects are reactions that would be expected to occur—at least in some people—because of the way a drug works in your body. For example, aspirin prevents heart attacks by interfering with the ability of your blood to clot. This also makes you more prone to bleed, so a bloody nose after a mild jolt is considered a predictable side effect of taking aspirin.

Over-dosage is a common cause of adverse reactions. Almost any drug will cause adverse effects if the dose is too high. An absolute overdose occurs when you take more than the recommended amount on the label. But someone who is extremely small and light can experience a relative overdose by following label instructions that are generally written for a person of average size.

Unpredictable Adverse Drug Reactions

Allergic reactions are caused by an immune response to a medication. The body erroneously recognizes the drug as a threat and attempts to destroy it.

Intolerance to a medication occurs when a drug produces its expected side effects at recommended doses. For example, most people will experience ringing in the ears if they take very high doses of aspirin, but people who are intolerant to aspirin will develop the problem on recommended doses.

Idiosyncratic reactions are rare, uncharacteristic and usually have nothing to do with the way the drug is supposed to work in the body. For example, African-American men and women occasionally develop a severe form of anemia after taking primaquine, an antimalarial medication.

The most common signs of an allergic drug reaction include:

Skin rashes: Typically, allergic drug rashes are red, raised and itchy, and appear on several areas of the body. When the reaction is caused by a topical medication, the rash will appear wherever the ointment or cream was applied, and it may also appear on the hand that applied the medication.

Hives (urticaria): These are raised welts that can appear anywhere on the body. They are not dangerous, but can cause serious discomfort because of itching (see pages 133-142 for more information about hives).

Angioedema: This is localized fluid accumulation in the skin (edema) that can cause significant swelling of the hands and feet, eyelids, lips and throat. Angioedema usually occurs in association with hives, but it may also occur alone (see pages 133-142 for more information about angioedema).

Other less common allergic drug reactions include the following:

Photosensitivity: A rash appears wherever the skin is exposed to the sun because of an interaction between the drug and the light rays. Exposure to direct sunlight is usually required, but this rash can also be triggered by artificial light. Rashes due to photosensitivity may be due to an allergy, or they can occur without involving the immune system.

Fixed drug eruption: This type of allergic reaction causes dark purple, round or oval spots to appear on the skin or inside the mouth. The spots may vary in size from just a few millimeters in diameter to more than 10 inches. A unique feature of this eruption is that the lesions always appear in the same locations every time the offending drug is taken.

Exfoliative dermatitis: This reaction causes superficial shedding of skin over the entire body (even the hair and nails may be lost). The skin all over the body becomes red and scaly. This reaction can be life-threatening, because it destroys the protective physical barrier that the skin normally provides.

Erythema multiforme: This is a rash that appears on the back of the hands and feet (sometimes on the palms and soles, also), and on the front of the legs and back of the arms (in some individuals, it may occur all over the body). The rash may be slightly itchy or painful, and is often accompanied by a headache and fever.

Stevens-Johnson syndrome: This condition resembles erythema multiforme, but typically produces much more tissue damage, especially in the mucous membranes that line the mouth, throat and some of the internal organs. In up to 5% of cases, the reaction is severe enough to cause death.

Reactions affecting internal organs: Allergic reactions to drugs are not confined to the skin. They can also affect the lungs (causing asthma or pneumonia); the blood (resulting in destruction of blood cells and anemia); and the liver and kidneys (interfering with normal function and causing tissue destruction).

Anaphylaxis: Drug allergy can also produce a life-threatening anaphylactic reaction, with a severe drop in blood pressure, swelling of the throat and difficulty breathing. Symptoms generally begin soon after the medication is taken (typically within about 30 minutes). If not treated quickly, typically by the injection of epinephrine, death can occur (see pages 172-174 for more information about anaphylaxis).

Diagnosing a Drug Allergy

In most cases, the diagnosis of a drug allergy is based on your medical history. When an adverse reaction occurs soon after a new drug has been started, it's logical to assume that the drug was responsible for the reaction. Just to be sure, your physician will want to know what other drugs you have been taking, including over-the-counter medications. If, for example, you are using antibiotics to cure an infection, and you're also taking aspirin to control a fever, either drug could be causing the reaction.

KEEPING A DRUG RECORD

Start and maintain a lifelong record of all medications you use. Ideally, this should be part of the overall medical record you keep at home for every family member. If you do not keep such a record, start one and include the following information for every drug you use, including over-the-counter products:

- Chemical (generic) and brand name of the drug
- Dosage (strength)
- If a prescription drug, prescribing doctor
- Reason for using the drug
- Number of doses prescribed or used
- Dates medication was taken
- Compliance (What percentage of the medication you were supposed to use did you actually take?)
- Results (Was the medication effective?)
- Adverse reactions (side effects, allergic reaction)

Laboratory tests have not been developed to diagnose or confirm most drug allergies. But your physician may recommend one of the following procedures to identify a drug allergy:

Skin testing: This test is performed by placing a small amount of the suspected medication under the skin and monitoring your body's response to it. It is helpful in identifying allergies to only a few drugs, including penicillin.

Provocative test dosing: This test, used uncommonly, relies on increasing doses of the suspected drug to determine how your body will react. The test begins with extremely small doses; gradually larger doses are given if the small doses don't cause allergic symptoms. It may be used to desensitize an individual to a drug so it can be used in medically appropriate circumstances, often in an intensive care unit.

The tests described above should only be done under a doctor's immediate supervision, and only in a medical setting where a severe reaction could be treated appropriately immediately.

Treating a Drug Allergy

When a drug allergy is diagnosed—or even suspected—the most important step is to discontinue the medication. Symptoms and physical changes usually reverse themselves once the drug is stopped, although it may take a week for that to happen.

Whenever you suspect that you are reacting adversely to a drug, call your physician immediately to discuss the problem. In almost all instances, the doctor will be able to prescribe an alternate medication to which you are not allergic.

ALLERGIES TO PENICILLIN

Perhaps the best known drug allergy is to penicillin. About 10 - 15% of people surveyed believe they are allergic to penicillin. In fact, experts think only about 2% of the treated population is truly allergic to penicillin.

The most common allergic reaction to penicillin is a rash. However, severe anaphylactic reactions also occur, and are thought to cause between 300 and 800 deaths in the United States every year.

The best thing to do if you think you are allergic to penicillin—and certainly if you have ever had a severe allergic reaction to it—is avoid it entirely. You should also avoid taking any antibiotics that are closely related to penicillin (most have names that end in -illin), such as ampicillin and amoxicillin, and you should be cautious in the use of a group of antibiotics called cephalosporins since people who are allergic to penicillin can react to cephalosporins as well. Additionally, you should wear a tag or bracelet that identifies you as being allergic to penicillin.

If you are taking several drugs at the same time, it may be difficult to determine which one is causing an allergic reaction. If the reaction is mild, your doctor may recommend that you discontinue only the most suspicious drug to see if your symptoms improve. (For example, if you have been taking blood pressure medication for many years and develop a rash several days after starting a course of penicillin, it makes sense to discontinue only the penicillin.) If there is no improvement after discontinuing a single drug, the next most likely drug can be stopped, and so on until the culprit is uncovered. If you are having a severe reaction, it may be necessary to stop all drugs at once, and then reintroduce them one at a time.

Occasionally, it may be necessary to take a medication to which you are allergic. If so, it may be possible to decrease your reaction to it through a process called desensitization (see *Provocative test dosing* on page 180).

Reducing Your Risk of Serious Drug Reactions

Here are some simple guidelines that will help you minimize your risk of a serious drug reaction in the future:

- Take medications only when they are absolutely necessary (even over-the-counter drugs and homeopathic medicines).

- Never take any medications to which you have a known allergy or to which you suspect you may be allergic, unless your physician can explain why there is no other alternative.

- Maintain a complete history at home of all the drugs you are currently taking or have used in the past (see box, *Keeping A Drug Record,* on page 179).

- Make sure that all physicians who care for you have a complete list of drugs to which you have had an allergic reaction. This will reduce the risk of an inadvertent prescription for the same drug later, or for a drug known to cross-react with it.

- Buy all of your medications (including over-the-counter drugs) at the same pharmacy. Be sure that the pharmacist maintains an up-to-date computerized "patient profile" on you. This should list every medication you are taking (including over-the-counter drugs) and every known allergy. This will reduce the risk of your receiving a drug to which you are allergic. It will also protect against your receiving two drugs at the same time that should not be taken together.

- If you have had any serious allergic reactions to drugs, wear a Medic Alert bracelet or pendant so you will not accidentally receive any of those drugs during an emergency situation when you are unable to communicate with the doctors.

Drugs that Frequently Cause Allergic Reactions

The risk of suffering a true allergic reaction is about 1 - 3% for most drugs. The list below includes some of the more commonly used drugs that have a known risk of triggering allergic reactions. (Please note that the following is in alphabetical order, not in order of risk, and does not include every drug known to cause allergic reactions.)

Type of Drug	Brand Name	Type of Drug	Brand Name
Antibiotics		*Antibiotics (cont'd)*	
aminoglycosides		cefonicid	Monocid ®
gentamicin	Garamycin ®	cefoperazone	Cefobid ®
streptomycin		cefotaxime	Claforan ®
cephalosporins		cefotetan	Cefotan ®
cefaclor	Ceclor ®	cefoxitin	Mefoxin ®
cefadroxil	Duricef ®	cefpodoxime	Vantin ®
cefamandole	Mandol ®	cefprozil	Cefzil ®
cefazolin	Ancef ®	ceftazidime	Ceptaz ®
	Kefzol ®		Fortaz ®
cefixime	Suprax ®		Tazicef ®
			Tazidime ®

Type of Drug	Brand Name
Antibiotics (cont'd)	
ceftibuten	Cedax ®
ceftizoxime	Cefizox ®
ceftriaxzone	Rocephin ®
cefuroxime	Ceftin ®
	Kefurox ®
	Zinacef ®
cephalexin	Keflex ®
	Keftab ®
chloramphenicol	Chloromycetin ®
ciprofloxacin	Cipro ®
clindamycin	Cleocin ®
erythromycin	Ery-Tab ®
ethambutol	Myambutol ®
griseofulvin	Fulvicin ®
	Grifulvin ®
	Grisactin ®
isoniazid	Rifamate ®
	Rifater ®
ketoconazole	Nizoral ®
metronidazole	Flagyl ®
miconazole	Monostat ®
nalidixic acid	NegGram ®
nitrofurantoin	Macrodantin ®
	Macrobid ®
penicillins	
amoxicillin	Amoxil ®
	Augmentin ®
ampicillin	Omnipen ®
	Unasyn ®
bacampicillin	Spectrobid ®
carbenicillin	Geocillin ®
mezlocillin	Mezlin ®
nafcillin	Unipen ®
penicillin G	Bicillin ®
penicillin V	Pen-Vee K ®
piperacillin	Pipracil ®
	Zosyn ®

Type of Drug	Brand Name
Antibiotics (cont'd)	
ticarcillin	Ticar ®
	Timentin ®
polymyxin B	Cortisporin ®
	Neosporin ®
	Polysporin ®
pyrazinamide	Rifater ®
rifampin	Rifadin ®
	Rifamate ®
	Rifater ®
sulfamethoxazole	Bactrim™
	Gantanol ®
	Septra ®
tetracyclines	
demeclocycline	Declomycin ®
doxycycline	Monodox ®
	Vibramycin ®
minocycline	Dynacin ®
	Minocin ®
	Vectrin ®
tetracycline	Achromycin ®V
trimethoprim	Bactrim™
	Proloprim ®
	Septra ®
	Trimpex ®
vancomycin	Vancocin ®
Anticoagulants	
heparin	
Anticonvulsants	
carbamazepine	Epitol™
	Tegretol ®
clonazepam	Klonopin ®
ethosuximide	Zarontin ®
phenobarbital	Acro-Lase ® Plus
	Bellatal™
	Donnatal ®
	Quadrinal™
phenytoin	Dilantin ®
valproic acid	Depakene ®

Type of Drug	Brand Name
Antidepressants	
monoamine oxidase inhibitors	
phenelzine	Nardil ®
tranylcy-promine	Parnate ®
tricyclic antidepressants	
amitriptyline	Elavil ®
	Etrafon ®
	Limbitrol ®
	Triavil ®
clomipramine	Anafranil ®
desipramine	Norpramin ®
imipramine	Tofranil ®
nortriptyline	Pamelor ®
protriptyline	Vivactil ®
Antipsychotics	
haloperidol	Haldol ®
Anxiety Medication	
meprobamate	Equagesic ®
	Equanil ®
	Miltown ®
Arrhythmia Medication	
digoxin	Lanoxin ®
procainamide	Procanbid™
quinidine	Quinaglute ®
	Quinidex Extentabs ®
Arthritis Medication	
gold salts	
auranofin	Ridaura ®
aurothioglucose	Solganal ®
gold sodium thiomalate	Myochrysine ®
penicillamine	Cuprimine ®
	Depen ®

Type of Drug	Brand Name
Aspirin and Non-steroidal Anti-inflammatory Drugs	
acetaminophen	Tylenol ®
diclofenac	Voltaren ®
diflunisal	Dolobid ®
etodolac	Lodine ®
ibuprofen	Advil ®
	Motrin ®
indomethacin	Indocin ®
ketoprofen	Orudis ®
	Oruvail ®
ketorolac	Toradol ®
mefenamic acid	Ponstel ®
nabumetone	Relafen ®
naproxen	Aleve ®
	Anaprox ®
	Naprelan ®
oxaprozin	Daypro ®
piroxicam	Feldene ®
sulindac	Clinoril ®
tolmetin	Tolectin ®
Blood Pressure Medication	
clonidine	Catapres ®
	Combipres ®
hydralazine	Hydra-Zide
methyldopa	Aldoclor ®
	Aldomet ®
	Aldoril ®
Chemotherapeutic Agents	
bleomycin	Blenoxane ®
busulfan	Myleran ®
cisplatin	Platinol ®
cyclophosphamide	Cytoxan ®
cytarabine	Cytosar-U ®
doxorubicin	Adriamycin ®
	Doxil ®
	Rubex ®

Type of Drug	Brand Name
Chemotherapeutic Agents (cont'd)	
melphalan	Alkeran ®
methotrexate	Rheumatrex ®
Diabetes Medication	
chlorpropamide	Diabinese ®
Diuretics	
ethacrynic acid	Edecrin ®
furosemide	Lasix ®
thiazide diuretics	
hydrochloro-thiazide	Aldactazide ®
	Aldoril ®
	Capozide ®
	Dyazide ®
	HydroDIURIL ®
	Hydropres ®
	Hyzaar ®
	Inderide ®
	Oretic ®
	Prinzide ®
	Timolide ®
	Vaseretic ®
	Zestoretic ®
	Ziac ®
chlorothiazide	Aldoclor ®
	Diupres ®
	Diuril ®
methy-clothiazide	Aquatensen ®
	Diutensen ®-R
	Enduron ®
triamterene	Dyazide ®
	Dyrenium ®
	Maxzide ®
Endometriosis Medication	
danazol	Danocrine ®
Enzymes	
asparaginase	
cymopapain	

Type of Drug	Brand Name
Enzymes (cont'd)	
chymotrypsin	
trypsin	
Gastrointestinal Reflux Medication	
metoclopramide	Reglan ®
Gout Medication	
allopurinol	Zyloprim ®
colchicine	ColBENEMID ®
Hormones	
insulin	Humulin ®
	Novolin ®
	Velosulin ®
Local Anesthetics	
bupivacaine	Sensorcaine ®
chloroprocaine	Nesacaine ®
etidocaine	Duranest ®
lidocaine	Xylocaine ®
Migraine Headache Medication	
ergotamine	Ergomar ®
	Wigraine ®
Myocardial Infarction	
papaverine	
streptokinase	Streptase ®
Osteoporosis Medication	
calcitonin	Miacalcin ®
Pain Medication	
opiates	
codeine	
fentanyl	
hydrocodone	Hycodan ®
	Lortab ®
	Vicodin ®
hydromorphone	Dilaudid ®
meperidine	Demerol ®
methadone	Dolophine ®
morphine	MS Contin ®
oxycodone	Percocet ®

Type of Drug	Brand Name
Pain Medication (cont'd)	
	Percodan ®
	Roxicet™
pentazocine	Talacen ®
	Talwin ®
propoxyphene	Darvocet ®
	Darvon ®
Parkinson's Disease Medication	
levodopa	Atamet ®
	Larodopa ®
	Sinemet ®

Type of Drug	Brand Name
Peptic Ulcer Medication	
ranitidine	Zantac ®
Stroke Medication	
ticlopidine	Ticlid ®
propoxyphene	Darvocet ®
	Darvon ®
Vaccines	
Influenza	
MMR (measles/mumps/rubella)	
Yellow Fever	

Chapter 10

Occupational Allergies

The workplace has always been a major source of allergic problems. In preindustrial times, most of these problems were triggered by occupational contact with proteins from animals and plants. But today, the development of thousands of new chemical compounds has dramatically increased the number of potential allergens and irritants to which workers are exposed. Not surprisingly, the number of people with occupational allergies has also dramatically increased. Their problems fall into three major categories: occupational asthma, allergic rhinitis and allergic contact dermatitis.

The range of work-related substances that can trigger allergies is extremely wide, and almost no occupation is completely free of problems. Every occupation has its own particularly troublesome allergens, each with its own typical pattern of reactions. Bakers, for example, are constantly exposed to several allergenic substances, including wheat protein, alpha amylase (a flour additive), cinnamon and storage mites. A study of 485 bakers revealed that 14.4% had rhinitis and 6.4% had asthma. Occupational exposure to allergens was thought to be responsible for two-thirds of the rhinitis and more than half of the asthma cases. Allergic contact dermatitis is also very common among bakers, probably due to alpha amylase exposure.

Hair dyes are the greatest problem for beauticians, causing many to suffer from allergic contact dermatitis. Carpenters commonly complain of allergic rhinitis, caused by inhaling wood dust, especially from the Western Red Cedar.

Unfortunately, occupational allergies are often misdiagnosed. Sometimes this occurs because sick workers and their physicians simply fail to consider the possibility that workplace allergens are responsible for the symptoms. And in some cases, the diagnosis of occupational allergy is considered, but erroneously eliminated because workers and their doctors fail to recognize the allergens at work. Allergens such as flour and garlic powder, for example, are not well-known as allergens. Even when the exposure to occupational allergens is obvious, physicians can be misled if the worker has been exposed for long periods of time without developing symptoms; unlike most other allergies, reactions to occupational allergens can take months or years to develop.

The type of allergic reaction a worker will experience depends on the specific allergen involved and the route of exposure. Inhaled allergens are most likely to trigger occupational asthma or rhinitis, while allergens that come in contact with the skin are most likely to trigger a skin reaction (dermatitis). While some workplace allergens can cause either skin disease or asthma (latex, for example), most produce one or the other, not both.

Some workplace allergens tend to trigger more severe reactions than others, but the extent and frequency of exposure will also determine the severity. For example, daily exposure to high concentrations of a normally mild allergen could trigger a much more severe reaction than infrequent exposure to small amounts of a normally powerful allergen. In general, the greater the exposure to any allergen, the more likely it is to produce disease and the more severe the disease is likely to be. However, sensitized workers usually respond to very small levels of allergens and even a minute exposure is capable of causing a problem.

Allergic Occupational Skin Disease

Of all occupational diseases, skin problems are by far the most common, accounting for about 30% of all work-related illnesses. But not all work-related skin problems are caused by allergies. In fact, the most frequent occupational skin disease is *irritant contact dermatitis*, which results from a direct physical injury to the skin by an irritating or toxic substance (such as a strong acid or lye). When dermatitis is the result of direct irritation, redness appears soon after contact with the responsible substance (especially when extremely irritating or corrosive substances are involved). In very severe cases, the skin may blister or actually slough off.

Only about 20% of occupational skin problems are actually the result of an allergic reaction to the chemical or substance. The rash that results (*allergic contact dermatitis*) is caused by a reaction of sensitized immune cells (lymphocytes). When allergy is responsible, the appearance of inflammation is usually delayed; the typical red, patchy rash appears about 12 to 48 hours after contact with the allergenic chemical or substance. In severe cases, blisters may be present and the skin may swell. The rash occurs only in areas that the allergen has contacted. (An allergic reaction to rubber gloves, for example, will usually affect the hands and forearms; hair dye will cause a rash on the scalp and the hands if gloves were not worn when the dye was applied.)

Irritant contact dermatitis and allergic contact dermatitis can be very difficult to tell apart from their appearance alone. Patch testing may help differentiate between the two. A patch containing the suspected chemical or substance is applied to a small area of skin, then examined after 48 hours, and again two days later. If the patch of skin shows signs of inflammation (redness or blisters, for example) which persist for several days, it suggests that the worker is allergic (irritative reactions typically subside in a few hours).

Treatment of Allergic Contact Dermatitis

Whatever the cause of contact dermatitis—irritant or allergy—the first step in managing the problem is to remove the offending substance and prevent all further contact with it. If contact cannot be avoided, the area affected should be immediately and thoroughly washed with plain water (mild soap may be used, if necessary, to remove oily substances). Another option is to wear cotton gloves.

Treatment of the rash is focused on reducing the inflammation and providing symptomatic relief. Topical corticosteroid creams are the first choice to combat the inflammation.

If an allergic contact rash is very extensive or it involves the face or genital area, systemic corticosteroid drugs (taken orally) will need to be used. Typically, these medications are prescribed for 5 to 10 days, starting with a higher dose that gradually tapers downward. Your doctor should be your guide on any medication you use for allergic contact dermatitis.

For symptomatic relief, cool, moist compresses can be applied direct-ly to the area of the rash. A soft, clean cloth (such as a handkerchief) should be soaked in cool water. This should be repeated 2-4 times a day for 10-15 minutes at a time. After compressing the area, it should be gently patted dry (not rubbed), and the steroid cream applied. Once the inflammation diminishes (which can take 3-4 days), the compresses can be discontinued and the steroid cream used alone. It may take two weeks for the rash to clear completely, although associated symptoms, such as itching, may subside more rapidly.

Oral antihistamines can control the itching associated with allergic contact dermatitis. In most cases, physicians will not use topical anti-histamine and antibiotic creams and ointments to treat an allergic rash.

COMMON OCCUPATIONAL CAUSES OF ALLERGIC SKIN REACTIONS

Occupation	Allergen
Aircraft assembly worker	Chromates, Epoxy resins, Synthetic rubber
Cashier	Nickel
Cement worker	Chromates
Construction worker	Chromates, Epoxy resins, Synthetic rubber
Dentist	Acrylics, Balsam of Peru, Epoxy resins, Glutaraldehyde, Gutta percha, Latex, Mercury
Electrician	Chromates, Epoxy resins, Synthetic rubber
Electroplating worker	Chromates, Nickel
Embalmer	Formaldehyde
Florist	Chrysanthemum, Poison ivy, Tulips
Gardener	Chrysanthemum, Poison ivy, Tulips
Hairdresser	Ammonium persulfate, Glycerol thioglycolate, Nickel, Paraphenylenediamine

Occupation	Allergen
Healthcare worker	Acrylics, Antibiotics, Carbamates, Formaldehyde, Glutaraldehyde, Latex, Mercaptobenzothiazole, Phenothiazines, Thiurams
Homemaker	Carbamates, Mercaptobenzothiazole, Thiurams
Insulation worker	Formaldehyde
Jeweler	Nickel
Laboratory worker	Formaldehyde
Mason	Carbamates, Mercaptobenzothiazole, Thiurams
Mechanic	P-Phenylenediamine
Mortician	Formaldehyde
Painter	Chromates, Epoxy resins, Synthetic rubber
Paper mill worker	Formaldehyde
Pharmacist	Acrylics, Antibiotics, Formaldehyde, Glutaraldehyde, Latex, Phenothiazines
Plastic worker	Epoxy resins
Printer	Chromates
Tanner	Chromates
Textile worker	Formaldehyde
Tire worker	P-Phenylenediamine
Veterinarian	Acrylics, Antibiotics, Formaldehyde, Glutaraldehyde, Latex, Phenothiazines
Wood worker	Wood dusts

Prevention of Allergic Contact Dermatitis

The most important thing you can do to treat this condition is to avoid the chemical or substance that is causing the problem. Sometimes protective clothing can be worn to prevent contact with it from occurring. In other cases, you must find a new agent to use in place of the one causing you trouble. Avoiding what you are allergic to will not only allow any skin reaction you have developed to heal, but will prevent new rashes from developing as well.

Occupational Asthma

The term *occupational asthma* refers to asthmatic changes that are triggered by exposure to irritants and allergens at work. It is estimated that 2-15% of all new asthma cases in the United States are triggered by occupational exposures. In some cases, asthma is the result of direct physical irritation of the airways by high levels of toxic substances (such as ammonia fumes or smoke). Other cases are truly allergic in nature, occurring only after a person has become sensitized to the allergen.

In many respects, occupational asthma behaves just like other forms of asthma, causing narrowing and irritability of the airways that results in wheezing and difficulty breathing. However, with occupational asthma, the symptoms typically begin within 10-20 minutes of arrival at work, and improve after the individual leaves the worksite for another location. Most people are free of symptoms (or their symptoms improve) on their days off and when on vacation. However, chronic exposure to some occupational allergens can result in chronic inflammation that does not improve until the worker has been away from the offending allergen for months or years.

The symptoms of irritant-induced asthma (wheezing, cough and difficulty breathing) do not require a period of sensitization and can begin very quickly after the toxic substance is first inhaled (usually within 24 hours). However, allergic asthma symptoms do not occur the first time you are exposed to an allergen in the workplace. First, you must become sensitized to the allergen, which requires one or more exposures to it. In fact, sensitization may take months or even years to occur. This long delay between the first exposure to allergens at work and the onset of symptoms can make it difficult to identify the actual cause of the problem.

COMMON OCCUPATIONAL CAUSES OF ASTHMA

At least 200 different agents in the workplace have been shown to cause asthma. Here is a list of some common offenders:

Occupation	Agent
Aircraft fitter	Triethylene tetramine
Agricultural worker	Cow dander
Angler	L. caesar larvae
Animal handler	Guinea pig, Mouse, Rabbit, Rat
Apple grower	Acarian
Aquarium keeper	Fish-feed
Baker	Buckwheat, Gluten, Fungal amylase, Fungal amyloglucosidade, Fungal hemicellulase, Flour
Bottle cap manufacturer	Polyvinyl chloride
Brewery worker	Hops
Butcher	Pig
Candy maker	Pectin
Carpenter	Wood dusts
Carpet manufacturer	Guar
Chemical worker	Anhydrides, Chloramine T
Chemist	Piperazine hydrochloride
Chicory grower	Chicory
Construction worker	Wood dusts
Dairy worker	Lactoserum
Decorator	Cocoon seed
Detergent industry worker	B. subtilis, Esperase
Diamond polisher	Cobalt
Dyer	Lanasol yellow 4G

Occupation	Agent
Egg producer	Egg protein
Electronics worker	Colophony
Entomologist	Butterflies, Moths
Farmer	Barn mite, Grain mite, Soybeans, Tetracholoroisophthalonitrile, Vicia sativa
Fish bait breeder	Bee moth
Fisherman	Cuttlefish, Red soft coral
Flight crew	Screw worm fly
Floor varnisher	Diisocyanate
Florist	Baby's breath
Flour handler	Lathyrus sativus, Mites, Parasites
Foam manufacturer	Urea formaldehyde
Food worker	Coffee bean, Garlic dust, Gluten
Foundry worker	Diisocyanate
Fur dyer	Paraphenylene diamine
Furniture maker	Wood dusts
Glove manufacturer	Latex
Grain elevator operator	Grain dust
Grain worker	Grain mite, Lesser mealworm
Grinder	Tungsten carbide
Hairdresser	Acacia, Henna, Karaya, Persulphate salts
Hard metal grinder	Cobalt
Healthcare worker	Latex, Psyllium
Honey processor	Honeybee
Horticulturist	Freesia, Paprika
Hospital worker	Formaldehyde, Glutaraldehyde, Hexachlorophene
Insulation installer	Urea formaldehyde
Janitorial worker	Chloramine T
Laboratory worker	Cockroaches, Crickets, Fruit flies, Laboratory animals, Locusts, Rats
Locksmith	Zinc fumes

Occupation	Agent
Longshoreman	Castor beans
Meat wrapper	Polyvinyl chloride
Metal plating industry worker	Nickel
Miller	Flour
Nurse	Cyanocrylates, Chlorhexidine, Ethylene dioxide, Latex, Methyl methacrylate
Oyster farmer	Hoya
Painter	Diisocyanate, Dimethyl ethanolamine
Paint store worker	Diisocyanate
Paper packer	Polyethylene
Pharmaceutical worker	Bromelin, Cephalosporins, Cimetidine, Egg lysosyme, Flaviastase, Hydralazine, Ipecacuanha, Methyl dopa, Opiate compounds, Pancreatin, Papain, Pepsin, Penicillins, Penicillamine, Phenylglycine acid chloride, Piperazine hydrochloride, Psyllium, Rose hips, Spiramycin, Tetracycline, Trypsin, Tylosin tartrate
Pharmacist	Isonicotinic acid hydrazide
Photographer	Ethylene diamine
Plant keeper	Weeping fig
Plastic manufacturer	Anhydrides, Azodicarbonamide, Diisocyanate, Trypsin
Plater	Chromium
Platinum refinery worker	Platinum
Plywood factory worker	Neurospora
Poultry worker	Chicken, Fowl mite, Lesser mealworm
Prawn processor	Prawn
Printer	Acacia, Chromium
Refrigeration worker	Freon
Resin manufacturer	Anhydrides, Urea formaldehyde
Rubber manufacturer	Azodicarbonamide, Diisocyanate
Rubber tire manufacturer	Tall oil
Sawmill worker	Wood dusts
Shellac handler	Ethylene diamine
Silk worker	Silkworm

Occupation	Agent
Ski manufacturer	3-DMAPA
Snow-crab processor	Crab
Solderer	Zinc fumes
Tanner	Casein, Chromium, Nickel
Tea processor	Herbal tea, Tea
Textile worker	Cibachrome brilliant scarlet 32, Drimaren brilliant blue K-BL, Drimaren brilliant yellow K-3GL
Tobacco manufacturer	Tobacco leaf
Tool setter	Anhydrides
Toy maker	Latex
Venipuncture technician	Tributyl tin oxide
Veterinarian	Mouse
Welder	Chromium, Nickel

Reprinted with permission. ©1994 *"Aetiological Agents in Occupational Asthma,"* *European Respiratory Journal.*

Diagnosing Occupational Asthma

The diagnosis of occupational asthma is sometimes easy—for example, when a person develops asthma shortly after starting a new job that involves working with well-known allergens. Unfortunately, the diagnostic process is usually not that simple. Many people simply aren't aware that they're working with allergenic substances, and their allergic reactions may not occur until months or years after their first contact with the allergens.

The key to success in diagnosing an occupational allergy is a thorough medical history and repeated physical examinations.

The medical history should include:

- A complete description of all chemicals, plants and animal substances with which you have come in contact at work for at least a year before the reaction occurred (see chart on pages 195-198 for a list of the most common offenders).

- A review of all previous jobs that might have put you in contact with any allergenic substances.

- A review of all symptoms, with special emphasis on when and where they occur. (Do you get worse at work and better at home? Do you feel well on your days off? Does anything aggravate your symptoms, such as exposure to cigarette smoke?) What, if anything, makes them better?

- Family history of allergy.

- Personal history of previous allergic reactions.

- All medications you are taking (especially any drugs you take to relieve allergic symptoms).

YOUR RIGHT TO KNOW ABOUT YOUR WORK ENVIRONMENT

You have a legal right to know about the chemicals you are exposed to at work. If you are concerned about any materials or chemicals that are present in your workplace, ask your employer for the *Material Safety Data Sheets* on those substances. Employers are required by the Occupational Safety and Health Administration (OSHA) to have this information available and to share it with employees on request. Checking the *Material Safety Data Sheets* for your workplace could provide you and your physician with valuable clues about the cause of any symptoms you are experiencing.

The physical examination is particularly useful when the lungs sound clear on days off, but wheezing is heard when the lungs are examined during a work shift or immediately afterward.

Other tests and procedures that can help in the diagnosis include the following:

- Chest x-rays can help identify (or exclude) other types of lung disease that could be causing the symptoms.

- Skin testing will be helpful if the list of suspected allergens is small, and if tests are available for the particular substances suspected (tests are not available for many occupational allergens).

- Blood testing may be helpful if the list of suspected allergens is small; but specific blood tests are not available for many occupational allergens.

- Pulmonary function tests measure your lung capacity and your ability to move air in and out of your lungs. Comparing the results of tests done before and after a work shift may reveal a significant difference caused by exposure to allergens at work. Your doctor may recommend performing these peak flow tests every two to four hours at work, and then when you're not at work.

- Bronchial response tests will reveal if the airways are overly irritable (a characteristic of asthma) by testing their response to the drug, methacholine. By comparing the results of tests done before and after work, your doctor can determine whether a significant difference exists when you're exposed to workplace allergens.

• Inhalation "challenge" or "provocation" tests can be performed when other testing has failed to identify the specific allergen (or allergens) that are causing the problem. These tests are performed by actually breathing the suspected allergens from work, and observing the response. Provocation testing should be performed by experts in occupational asthma and only in medical settings where emergency treatment can be administered immediately in the event of a severe asthmatic reaction.

Treatment of Occupational Asthma

The most important step in the treatment of occupational asthma is to prevent all further exposure to the offending allergen, and the sooner this is done, the better. Workers whose exposures are ended quickly after the onset of their symptoms usually get better quickly; those who continue to be exposed can develop severe asthma that persists for years after leaving work.

Among the ways to prevent further exposures:

• Develop alternative procedures at work to isolate workers from exposure to the allergen (such as masks, other physical barriers and improved ventilation systems).

• Identify alternative substances that can be substituted for the offending allergen.

• Reassign allergic employees to other positions in the company.

• Seek work elsewhere. (People who must leave their jobs because of work-related allergies may qualify for disability benefits.)

The medical treatment of occupational asthma is identical to the treatment of asthma that is unrelated to work. For a complete description, see Chapter 11.

Occupational Rhinitis

The inhaled allergens that trigger asthmatic reactions can also cause the onset of allergic rhinitis, producing nasal congestion, itchiness, sneezing and a runny nose. Some workers may suffer from both conditions at the same time, while others are affected by only one or the other.

ARE YOUR ALLERGIES RELATED TO WORK?

You should suspect that workplace allergens could be responsible for your asthma, rhinitis or dermatitis if you answer "yes" to some of the following questions:

- Do your symptoms occur only at work or worsen when you are at work?

- Do your symptoms improve after you leave work?

- Do your symptoms get better over the weekend or when you are on vacation?

- Do your symptoms improve if your assignment at work is temporarily changed?

- Do people with whom you work suffer similar symptoms?

- Do you work in one of the high-risk occupations listed on the charts in this chapter?

- Does your work bring you into contact with any of the high-risk substances listed on the charts in this chapter?

- Have you ever had an allergic reaction to chemicals or other work-related substances in the past?

Rhinitis, as with occupational asthma, may be the result of a direct physical injury by toxic inhalants (such as ammonia fumes), or it may be allergic in origin. The treatment for occupational rhinitis is the same as for rhinitis due to other causes. The same approach is employed to prevent further episodes of rhinitis as is used for occupational asthma.

Latex Allergies in Healthcare Workers

The AIDS epidemic has dramatically increased the use of latex gloves by all healthcare professionals and their assistants, and this has significantly increased the number of workers who are sensitized to latex. (It is estimated that 10-15% of all healthcare workers are now sensitized.) Vinyl gloves are an acceptable alternative for people who are allergic to latex. (Vinyl is a synthetic substance that contains no proteins.) But latex is still present in many other medical products that must be avoided—or used with great caution—by sensitized healthcare personnel (and any patients who are sensitized). These products include:

Adhesive bandages and tape	Esophageal dilators
Anesthesia masks	Esophageal protective covers
Bandages for burns	Eyedropper bulbs
Bite blocks	Face masks with elastic bands
Blood pressure cuffs	Feeding tubes
Breathing circuits	Finger cots
Catheters	Gloves (examination and surgical)
Cervical caps	Hemodialyzers
Cervical dilators	Hot water bottles
Dental dams	Injection adapters
Elastic bandages	Instrument mats
Electrode pads	IV injection ports
Endotracheal tubes	Nasopharyngeal airways

Orthodontic elastics	Syringe stoppers
Prophy cups	Tooth protectors
Rubber sheeting or pillows	Tourniquets
Rubber stoppers	Ultrasound covers
(for medicine bottles)	Urine bags and straps

Sick Building Syndrome

Over the last several decades, conservation-minded architects and engineers have changed the way buildings are designed in order to make them more energy-efficient. In essence, the buildings have been made "tighter," with windows that can't be opened and air that is constantly recirculated. This minimizes the amount of energy needed to run heaters in the winter and air conditioners during the summer.

Unfortunately, it has also created a new problem referred to as "sick building syndrome." The symptoms of this syndrome include headache, irritation of the eyes, nose and throat, and fatigue. People may also experience nausea, dizziness, and tightness or burning in the chest. Symptoms typically begin shortly after entering the building and are relieved soon after leaving.

It is believed that sick building syndrome occurs because inadequate amounts of fresh outside air are taken into the ventilation system, which allows chemicals and other contaminants to build up indoors, ultimately reaching levels that can cause symptoms in some people. Most experts believe that symptoms are the result of the accumulation of several different contaminants in the air at the same time. Thus far, no specific chemicals or contaminants have been proven to cause symptoms, but the leading suspects include:

- Formaldehyde, which is present in, and slowly evaporates from, a wide range of construction materials including plywood, particle board and some insulation materials
- Vapors from chemicals used in photocopiers and other office equipment
- Fumes from cleaning agents and solvents
- Tobacco smoke
- Molds/fungi
- Cooking gas fumes and aerosolized food particles

The treatment for sick building syndrome is to correct the source of the problem. Introducing more fresh air into the ventilation system and increasing the ventilation rate inside the building will usually eliminate the problem. Once the building is "cured," the symptoms of the people living and working in it should disappear.

Multiple Chemical Sensitivity

"Multiple chemical sensitivity" is a catch phrase for a controversial condition that makes its "victims" believe they are allergic to almost every modern chemical. These people complain of a wide array of symptoms ranging from headaches, joint pain and diarrhea to weakness, nausea and fatigue.

The diagnosis or even the existence of multiple chemical sensitivity is very controversial, because the symptoms tend to be vague, there are usually no consistent or objective physical abnormalities associated with the condition, and standard laboratory tests reveal no abnormalities of the immune system (or any other system). As a result, most allergy experts are skeptical that the disease actually exists.

Some physicians believe that multiple chemical sensitivity syndrome is psychological in nature, because of recent studies which show that people with this condition react to certain stimuli in the same manner as people with panic disorders or other psychiatric disorders. A small group of physicians who call themselves "clinical ecologists" believe that there is a physical basis for this disorder. Their usual recommendation to patients is to avoid contact with all modern chemicals, a difficult action that can involve considerable isolation and expense—and has no scientific basis.

Chapter 11

Asthma & Allergies

Even if you don't have asthma, you probably know someone who does. About 15 million Americans suffer from this chronic respiratory disease. That's more people than the entire population of Florida or Illinois! Yet people with asthma must feel as though they're struggling alone as they wheeze and strain just to take their next breath. Their chest becomes congested and tight. Their respiration becomes rapid and causes a wheezing sound or a persistent cough. Some people with asthma have compared their plight to trying to breathe through a straw filled with cotton. As they struggle for one breath, then another, they may become panicky, which can make their symptoms even worse.

Although this is a book about allergies, not asthma, the fact is that asthma and allergies are often intertwined. Allergies are one of the main triggers of asthma episodes. For that reason, this chapter may be particularly relevant if you or a family member have asthma. Although we won't cover the subject comprehensively, we'll describe what asthma is, what happens when an asthma episode occurs, how allergies contribute to asthma and resources you can turn to for more information.

What is Asthma?

The word "asthma" comes from the Greek term for breathlessness or panting. The disease is characterized by two major physiological problems:

- Chronic, underlying inflammation of the airways (or bronchial tubes)
- Muscle spasms that squeeze or tighten these airways

Before we really understood asthma, this disease was often labeled as a psychosomatic disorder. People with asthma were told that their illness was "all in your head," and that they didn't have a "real" disease. This notion became commonplace because the bronchial spasms and difficult breathing tended to worsen at times of psychological stress.

We now know that—although stress can aggravate the condition—inflammation of the airways is the real problem in people with asthma. This inflammation in the walls of the smaller bronchial tubes narrows the passages through which air must flow. It also makes the airways much more irritable and susceptible to muscular spasms that can narrow the passages even further.

In fact, the airways of people with asthma are *constantly* inflamed, even when they are not wheezing and having difficulty breathing. This inflammation occurs in response to several physical stimuli, including exposure to allergens that are inhaled, and it narrows the airways by thickening their walls and filling their passages with mucus. The inflammation can actually be observed using devices called fiberoptic bronchoscopes, which allow doctors to look directly into the lungs.

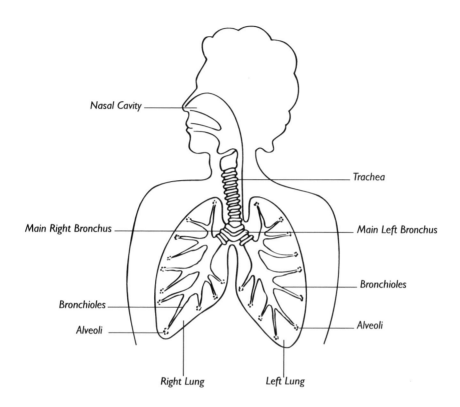

Nasal Cavity

Trachea

Main Right Bronchus

Main Left Bronchus

Bronchioles

Bronchioles

Alveoli

Alveoli

Right Lung

Left Lung

The branching system of airways permits air to pass deeply into the lungs to reach the tiny air sacs where oxygen is absorbed into the bloodstream and carbon dioxide is eliminated. The trachea, the tube that leads from the throat, divides into two main branches called bronchi, which channel air into each lung. The bronchi divide repeatedly to form progressively smaller tubes called bronchioles. The very smallest bronchioles terminate in collections of tiny air "sacs" called alveoli, which contain blood vessels (capillaries) within their thin walls. This is the place where oxygen from the air is absorbed into the bloodstream, and carbon dioxide from the blood is eliminated. In people with asthma, the flow of air through the bronchioles may be obstructed by inflammation or muscle spasm— both of which narrow the opening through which air must pass.

Only in recent years have we known about the continuous presence of this inflammation—and the crucial role it plays in asthma. As a result of this new knowledge, the treatment of asthma has changed dramatically. The foundation of all asthma therapy now involves the use of anti-inflammatory medications to control this aspect of the disease.

What Happens During an Asthma Episode?

Until asthma-related inflammation was clearly identified, physicians believed that muscle spasms in the walls of the airways ("bronchospasms") were the primary problem in an asthma episode. And, in fact, people with asthma do experience spasm and constriction of the smooth muscle tissue that surrounds their breathing passages. However, we now know that this constriction is secondary to the

ASTHMA: A FAMILY AFFAIR

Asthma often runs in families. More than two-thirds of people with asthma have a parent, a brother or a sister who has the disease. However, some people with asthma have no family members with it; conversely, a strong family history doesn't guarantee that you'll get asthma, although it will increase the likelihood.

Researchers are currently looking for the gene(s) that may increase your chances of having asthma. But keep in mind that you only inherit the *tendency* to have asthma, which is no guarantee that you will develop the disease. The incidence of asthma is on the increase, and factors other than heredity—such as the environment—also appear to play an important role in this medical condition.

underlying inflammation. The spasms are particularly likely to occur when the inflammation intensifies, or when these people are exposed to physically irritating stimuli such as tobacco smoke or noxious fumes, or after exposure to allergens to which they are sensitized.

As the smooth muscles in the walls of the breathing tubes contract, the diameter of the airway is narrowed, making it harder for air to flow into and out of the lungs. This narrowing also contributes to the wheezing sound and shortness of breath that are associated with asthma. Sometimes, the terms "twitchy" and "airway hypersensitivity" are used to describe the increased irritability of the breathing passages, the increased tendency for muscle spasms to occur, and the overreaction of the airways to external irritants and allergens.

Controlling the underlying inflammation in the airways is the key to successful therapy for asthma. Because the inflammatory process is chronic and ongoing, the treatment to control it must be constant and ongoing, also. If the initial breathing difficulties that inflammation causes are ignored or treated only symptomatically (with medications that dilate the airways but do nothing about the inflammation), the stage is set for severe—even life-threatening—episodes that can occur if muscle spasms narrow the airways even further.

During an asthma episode, when the respiratory tract is particularly inflamed and having spasms, people with asthma may say that it hurts just to breathe. Each time they exhale, they will have difficulty blowing out air from the lungs. Even though the chest cavity is filled with air, the narrowed respiratory tubes make normal breathing difficult, and wheezing or coughing can occur. Straining to exhale, some people with asthma say they feel as though they are suffocating or drowning.

The intensity of symptoms can vary from mild to severe, as can the frequency of asthma episodes. Some people have symptoms virtually every day. Others experience them only occasionally, and even then only during certain times of the year. Asthma symptoms (particularly coughing) tend to worsen at night and early morning. Some episodes develop very suddenly; more episodes come on gradually. Early warn-

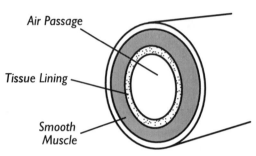

Figure 1: In a healthy lung, the small airways (bronchioles) are wide open and air can pass freely through them. The smooth muscle in the walls of the bronchioles is relaxed, and the tissue that lines the airways is free of inflammation.

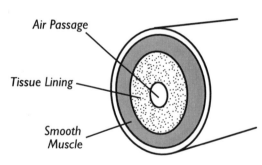

Figure 2: In a person with untreated asthma, the inner lining of the bronchioles becomes inflamed and thickened, which causes narrowing of the central air passage.

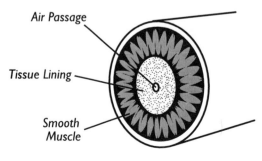

Figure 3: When inflammation is present, the airways become irritable, and the smooth muscle in the walls of the bronchioles is more susceptible to spasm. When the spasms occur, the opening in the air passage is narrowed down even more, and the flow of air may be "choked off" to dangerously low levels.

ing signs may be chest tightness, coughing and fatigue. As important as it is to directly treat these symptoms, unless the underlying inflammmation is aggressively treated as well, asthma complications—even potentially life-threatening ones—can develop.

Allergies & Your Asthma Episodes

Asthma episodes don't just come out of nowhere. They can be traced back to factors that intensify the underlying inflammation, causing an episode of wheezing, chest tightness and increased mucus production. The primary culprit is allergens. Among children with asthma, 80% have allergies; about half of adults with asthma are allergic.

If you have allergies, your immune system reacts to substances that, for most people, are completely harmless. As you've read earlier in this book, these include pollen, mold spores, house dust mites and animal dander. Upon exposure to these allergens, your immune system releases chemicals intended to fight off the invaders, but in people with asthma, this intensifies the inflammation that already exists in the respiratory system.

Although seasonal and household allergens are by far the most common agents that can induce asthmatic episodes, so can other types of allergies. For example, food allergies (such as to eggs, milk, wheat and peanuts) can occasionally provoke an asthma episode, especially in very young children; in cases like these, asthmatic symptoms usually occur a short time after the offending food is consumed.

Keep in mind that not everyone with asthma has allergies, or vice versa. Even if you do have both asthma and allergies, your episodes of asthma could be set off by factors other than allergies. In fact, many asthma episodes occur independent of allergies. In people with asthma, the interplay between allergens and certain other factors can make the responses even more problematic; for example, if your airways are already inflamed by ragweed in the middle of August, the added exposure to any of the following factors can make your asthmatic symptoms even worse:

Viral infections. If you have the common cold, bronchitis, a sore throat, the flu, a sinus infection, bronchiolitis or RSV (respiratory syncytial virus) infection, it can cause increased airway hyperreactivity and asthmatic symptoms.

Pollution. The hyperresponsive airways of a person with asthma can act up in the presence of pollutants, such as cigarette smoke, ozone and sulfur dioxide in the air. Smoke from charcoal grills and wood stoves can also be problematic for people with asthma, as can fumes from strong smelling chemicals such as paint, gasoline, perfumes and scented soaps.

Drugs. About 5 - 10% of adults with asthma will experience a worsening of their symptoms after taking aspirin or certain other drugs classified as non-steroidal anti-inflammatory agents (for example, ibuprofen and ketoprofen).

Industrial and occupational agents. On the job, you may encounter many substances that can provoke or intensify asthmatic episodes; they include various gases, vapors, and organic and inorganic dusts, often encountered in industrial settings.

Weather conditions. Your airways can become irritated by strong, dry winds, temperature shifts, cold air, and alterations in barometric pressure or humidity levels, such as occur during thunderstorms and other severe weather conditions.

The Right Diagnosis & Treatment

Asthma can't be cured. However, with proper treatment, asthma episodes can be effectively and safely managed, or even prevented.

The first step in getting the right therapy is to have your doctor make a proper diagnosis of the condition. Particularly if allergies are responsible for exacerbating asthma, you can help in this diagnostic process by letting your doctor know when asthma symptoms appear or become worse, such as during exposure to particular allergens. Use the *Asthma History* chart that follows to help in this process.

ASTHMA HISTORY

• What symptoms do I have?

     ___ Wheezing   ___ Coughing

     ___ Increased mucus production ___ Shortness of breath

     ___ Labored breathing   ___ Faster breathing

     ___ Chest tightness   ___ Distension of the chest

• When do my asthma symptoms most often occur?

     ___ Daytime   ___ Nighttime   ___ At home   ___ At work

     ___ During exercise ___ During particular activities

                        (such as cutting the lawn, gardening)

• Do my symptoms occur during certain seasons of the year? Yes ___ No ___

If yes, what season(s)? _____

_____

_____

- My symptoms seem to start when I'm exposed to the following
  substances or conditions:

___ Pollen	___ Colds, other infections
___ Grass, ragweed	___ Temperature changes
___ Molds	___ Chemicals/fragrances/fumes
___ Classroom environment	___ House dust
___ Tobacco smoke	___ Outdoor pollution
___ Fireplace smoke	___ Workplace environment

___ Foods (such as _____)

___ Pets (such as_____)

- How often do these symptoms occur?

___ Every day	___ Several times a month
___ More than twice weekly	___ Less than once a month

Once a diagnosis is made, your doctor may prescribe one or more
medications, including:

- **Long-term-control drugs,** which are prescribed to gain and maintain control of chronic or persistent asthma. These medications are
  sometimes called *preventers* or *prophylactic* drugs, and include daily
  medications such as cromolyn sodium, nedocromil sodium, inhaled
  and oral corticosteroids, theophylline and leukotriene modifiers.

Also included is the long-acting bronchodilator, Serevent®; however, it should not be used alone as a chronic medication, because it does not treat the underlying inflammation that accompanies asthma.

- **Quick-relief drugs,** which are prescribed to treat acute symptoms and episodes. They are sometimes called *relievers* or *rescue* medications, and include bronchodilators such as short-acting beta agonists, anticholinergics and corticosteroids.

Use all medications exactly the way your physician recommends. For many people, that means taking anti-inflammatory drugs every day, even when symptoms are not present. In addition, your doctor may also prescribe medications that temporarily dilate the airways. Although these drugs may provide dramatic temporary relief of wheezing and difficult breathing, they do not correct the underlying inflammation and should not be used as a substitute for anti-inflammatory medications. Your doctor may also prescribe medications for your allergies. Follow your doctor's guidelines for the use of every drug that is prescribed.

Special Issues in Childhood Asthma

Asthma is one of the most common chronic diseases that affect youngsters, and it causes substantial school absenteeism. About five million children under 18 years old in the U.S. have asthma. The prevalence of the disease is on the rise, as are the number of hospitalizations, particularly in preschool-age youngsters. Childhood asthma isn't something to be taken lightly.

Remind your child with asthma that he or she is no different than any other youngster, except for having a disease that's very treatable. If

MANAGING ASTHMA IN SCHOOL

The teachers and other staff personnel at your child's school need to know how to handle both everyday situations and emergencies related to your child's asthma. Share with them the following information, provided by The Asthma & Allergy Foundation of America.

WHAT TO LOOK FOR:

- Anxious look
- Stooped body posture
- Perspiring (diaphoresis)
- Rapid respirations (greater than 25-30 per minute at rest)
- Painful breathing
- Retractions (a concave appearance of the chest as the child struggles to breathe)
- Nasal flaring
- Nausea/vomiting
- Fatigue
- Decreased peak flow value (if a peak flow meter is used at school to monitor your child's status)

WHAT TO LISTEN FOR:

- Complaints of chest tightness
- Persistent coughing
- Irregular breathing
- Abnormal breath sounds (decreased or absent breath sounds; wheezing; rattling sounds while breathing)
- Prolonged expiration
- Rapid heart rate

WHAT TO DO IN AN ASTHMA CRISIS AT SCHOOL:

• Review the student's current medications and emergency medications.

• Have the student sit upright and check his breathing with a peak flow meter if possible.

• Administer prescribed medication by inhaler. (Medication should be inhaled slowly and fully.)

• Administer medication by nebulizer if prescribed.

• Reassure the student and attempt to keep him calm and breathing slowly and deeply.

• Student should respond to the treatment within 15-20 minutes. Recheck with a peak flow meter.

• If there is no change, or if the student's breathing becomes worse, contact the parent immediately and call for emergency help.

SEEK IMMEDIATE EMERGENCY CARE IF THE STUDENT HAS ANY OF THE FOLLOWING:

• Coughs constantly

• Is unable to speak in complete sentences without taking a breath

• Has lips, nails and mucous membranes that are gray or blue

• Demonstrates severe retractions and/or nasal flaring

• Is vomiting persistently

• Has 50% reduced peak flow reading

• Has a pulse greater than 120 per minute

• Has respirations greater than 30 per minute

• Is severely restless

• Shows no improvement after 15-20 minutes

your child is school-age, it is essential that you discuss the disease with school personnel, including your youngster's teacher and the school nurse. Your child may have to take medications at school, which will require that the staff become fully informed, and that you fill out treatment authorization forms that will be kept on file in the school office. Schedule a meeting with the school personnel, in which you should cover the following issues:

- Describe the medications that you will be sending to school with your child, and when they must be taken. Be sure you clearly differentiate between long-term-control and quick-relief drugs, and the circumstances under which each is to be given. Communicate your doctor's instructions on whether your child should carry the medication (like an inhaler) with him or her, or whether it should be kept in the nurse's office. Make certain the teacher and nurse are on the alert for and can recognize the wheezing and other symptoms that require administration of "rescue" medication. Let them know if your child will need help in administering the drug. Alert them to any side effects associated with these medications, particularly those (such as drowsiness, restlessness) that could interfere with your child's classroom performance. Put all of this information in writing—including the names of medications, the times of day they should be taken and the dose—and give a copy of it to the teacher and the nurse.

- Describe the allergens and irritants that may lead to asthmatic episodes in your child, and request that they be removed from your child's environment whenever possible. These may include classroom animals (gerbils, guinea pigs, rats), pollinating plants, certain chemicals, mold spores, cockroaches and chalk dust.

- Discuss any physical limitations that your doctor has placed upon your child, and/or the medications that he or she needs to take before physical activity. (Despite widely held beliefs to the contrary, all children with asthma can participate in P.E. classes when they are properly treated for their disease.)

- Talk with school officials and your doctor about what to do in an emergency—that is, if your child is having severe breathing problems and requires immediate medical attention. Your school should have phone numbers where both you and your child's physician can be reached.

Asthma Resources

You can also obtain additional information about asthma from the resources listed below.

The Asthma & Allergy Foundation of America
1125 15th Street NW, Suite 502
Washington, DC 20005
(800) 7-ASTHMA
www.aafa.org

American Academy of Allergy, Asthma and Immunology
611 E. Wells Street
Milwaukee, WI 53202
(800) 822-2762
www.aaaai.org

American College of Allergy, Asthma and Immunology
85 West Algonquin Road, Suite 550
Arlington Heights, IL 60005
(800) 842-7777
http://allergy.mcg.edu

National Jewish Medical and Research Center
1400 Jackson Street
Denver, CO 80206
Lung Line: (800) 222-LUNG
www.njc.org

American Lung Association
1740 Broadway
New York, NY 10019
(212) 315-8700
www.lungusa.org

National Asthma Education and Prevention Program
National Heart, Lung and Blood Institute
P.O. Box 30105
Bethesda, MD 20824
(301) 251-1222
www.nhlbi.nih.gov

Allergy and Asthma Network/Mothers of Asthmatics, Inc.
2751 Prosperity Avenue, Suite 150
Fairfax, VA 22031
(800) 878-4403 or (703) 641-9595

Chapter 12

Getting the Most Out of Your Doctor Visits

You now have the information and tools you need to manage your allergies successfully. You have learned many preventive steps to avoid—or at least minimize—exposure to the allergens that trigger your reactions. And when it's impossible to completely avoid the allergens you are sensitive to, you now know which treatments are available and appropriate for controlling allergic symptoms.

The most important thing you should have learned from reading this book is that no matter what your experience has been in the past, there is no longer any reason why you must suffer from allergies or let allergy symptoms "get you down." The key to managing your allergy problem is a strong partnership with your physician.

In this chapter, we will show you how to create that partnership, and how to get the most out of it. If you do not currently have a doctor who is dealing with your allergies, you'll learn how to find one. Or, if your current physician has not been able to help you with your allergy symptoms, we'll tell you how to find a specialist who may be able to. You'll learn how preparing in advance for your visits with the doctor can help you get more out of them. We'll advise you about which questions you should be prepared to answer, and how to get your own questions answered before you leave the doctor's office. These are all important steps in forming an effective partnership with your physician—one that will put you in control of your allergies.

Selecting a Doctor

If allergies are a problem, and you don't have a doctor who is working with you on solutions, it's time to find one. The best place to start is with the doctor who provides your primary care (most commonly an internist for adults, a pediatrician for children, or a family physician for children and adults). Most primary care physicians are familiar with and prepared to treat uncomplicated allergy problems.

If a primary care physician is treating your allergies successfully, there should be no need for you to see a specialist, unless problems develop that require consultation. For example, you may need to see a specialist if the treatments prescribed by your personal physician fail to relieve your symptoms, or if medical disorders (such as sinusitis, ear problems or asthma) develop while you are under treatment. With those conditions, it is helpful to consult with a Board-certified allergy-immunology specialist (usually referred to as an "allergist"). These specialists first trained as internists or pediatricians, completed a formal, two- or three-year postgraduate allergy training program at an accredited institution, and then proved their competence by passing a test administered by the American Board of Allergy and Immunology.

No matter what kind of physician you choose—generalist or specialist—it's essential that the doctor be interested in your total well-being, willing to devote whatever time is necessary to identify the offending allergens and treat you properly, and that he or she takes the problem of allergies seriously. As strange as it may sound, some physicians regard allergic symptoms as a minor inconvenience and therefore give allergy-related complaints a low priority in their practice. Given the already rushed conditions in today's managed healthcare environment, a physician who makes light of allergy problems makes it extremely difficult (if not impossible) for those with allergies to get the care they need. It may also mean that their allergic problem will not be diagnosed correctly.

Preparing for Your Appointment with the Doctor

Surveys show that many patients are dissatisfied with the outcome of their visits to the doctor, and the problem is likely to get worse as cost-cutting measures force physicians to spend less and less time with their patients. Usually, it's the doctor who gets blamed for the problem, and—sometimes—that's appropriate. But it's important to remember that patients bear some responsibility for the success of their doctor visits. As we pointed out earlier, successful treatment depends on a strong partnership between you and your doctor.

Here are a few ideas that will help you get your allergy-related problems solved when you're visiting the doctor:

- Prepare ahead of time for the "routine" questions that doctors almost always ask. If it's the first time you're seeing the doctor about allergies, expect to be asked for the information on pages 230-232; if it's a follow-up visit, you can expect to provide information like that beginning on page 232. Preparing your answers ahead of time—and in writing—will speed up the doctor's history-taking process, leaving more time for you to get your own questions answered by the doctor.

- Prepare your own list of questions—in writing—for the doctor. Having a written list makes it much less likely that you'll leave the doctor's office with some of your own questions unanswered. Try to list only the most important questions. Hand the questions to your doctor at the beginning of your visit.

- If you are making your first visit to a new physician, and you've been treated previously by other doctors for allergy problems, bring a copy of your past medical records and x-rays with you (or ask your previous doctors to send a copy of your records directly to your new doctor). This might save you from having to repeat some of the tests that have already been performed.

- Bring a list of all the medications you have taken in the past or are currently using. If you are not sure which drugs you have taken, ask your previous physician or your pharmacist to help you compile a list. If you do not know the names of drugs you are currently using, bring the medications with you in their original packaging.

What to Expect in the Doctor's Office

The first—and, often, the most important—step in the doctor's evaluation of your problem with allergies is a medical history. Allergy specialists say they are able to determine whether an allergy exists in almost 90% of the patients they see just on the basis of a careful medical history. For example, someone who has symptoms that get worse on workdays, improve on days off and disappear on vacations is almost certainly allergic to something in the workplace.

First, the doctor will want to take a general medical history, which will cover all of the important medical events in your life—not just the problems related to allergy. Then, a detailed allergy history will be taken. Your doctor may ask for more (or less) information than appears on the list on pages 230-232, depending on the unique features of your particular case.

After reviewing your medical history, the doctor will need to perform a complete medical examination, with special attention paid to your skin, eyes, nose, ears, throat and chest. (If you have already had a general physical exam by another physician, this examination may be limited to the particular areas related to your symptoms.) Typically, the doctor will examine the eyes and inside of the nose for signs of inflammation, swelling and discoloration. The ears will be examined to see if there are signs of fluid in the middle ear. The lungs will be examined for any signs of asthma, and the skin will be examined for evidence of eczema or allergic reactions.

Depending on what is learned during the medical history and found on physical examination, an allergy specialist may perform specific tests to confirm the general diagnosis of allergy and to identify the specific allergens that are causing reactions. These diagnostic tests include skin testing and blood tests (RAST), which are described in Chapter 4.

Once the diagnosis of allergy is made and the specific allergens causing your reaction have been identified, your doctor will help you develop strategies for managing the problem and eliminating your symptoms. Those strategies will depend on whether your allergies are seasonal or year-round; whether the offending allergens are primarily indoors or outdoors; and on the degree to which you are able to modify your life-style to reduce your exposure to these allergens.

The ideal strategy, of course, involves complete avoidance of the allergens that trigger your reactions. If you can avoid them completely, nothing further will be needed, because your allergic reactions will cease. Your doctor will identify the allergens you need to avoid, and will tell you what key actions are necessary to accomplish this goal. You will find detailed preventive strategies for all of the major allergens throughout this book.

When complete avoidance of allergens cannot be achieved, your doctor will help you develop a strategy for reducing and managing symptoms through the use of medication. If your symptoms occur only rarely, you'll be advised to use drugs only when they're needed. If your symptoms are present for long periods of time (for example, throughout a long pollen season), you'll be shown how to best use the medications for your condition.

If you are able to obtain relief from over-the-counter antihistamines without getting drowsy, your doctor will probably recommend that you continue their use. If they fail to relieve your symptoms, or they make you too drowsy to function effectively, the doctor is likely to recommend that you switch to one of the nonsedating medications. If you are good at remembering to take medications, your doctor may give you a choice of pills or nasal sprays, which must be taken or used several times a day. If remembering to take medicine multiple times a day is difficult for you, the doctor will probably suggest using a medication that only requires one dose a day. If you (or your child) can't swallow pills, the doctor can prescribe or recommend a medication in syrup form.

If you are at risk for an anaphylactic reaction that can create a potentially life-threatening situation, your doctor will probably advise that you always carry an emergency epinephrine kit with you. This kit will contain an automatic injector that enables you to administer the drug to yourself if danger signs appear. (For more information on these emergency kits, see pages 172-174.)

The key to success is working with your doctor to develop an allergy management program that is individualized to meet your particular needs. Before leaving your doctor's office, it is essential that you completely understand the prevention strategies that the doctor has recommended. If medications have been recommended or prescribed, be sure that you know precisely what dose the doctor wants you to use, and how often you should take it. Ask the doctor what side effects can occur with the medications you will be using, and what you should do if they appear.

In addition, determine what the doctor would like you to do in an emergency. Fortunately, such emergencies are rare, but it's important to be prepared for prompt action if they do occur. Have the doctor tell you which symptoms would require you to call 911. Identify the hospital emergency room that is preferred by your doctor, and know when to go there. And find out how best to contact the doctor when you have questions or need help quickly. The best time to learn this practical information is before you need to use it.

Finally, learn what to expect in the future. What kind of relief can you expect from your medication and how soon can you expect it? What should you do if you don't get the expected relief? How does the doctor plan to handle your follow-up care? How often will you need to be seen in the office? Under what conditions should you call for an earlier appointment? Knowing the answers to all of these questions *before* you leave the doctor's office will leave you with fewer questions to concern you later on. Having these answers will also leave you in better control of your allergies.

Taking an active role in the management of your allergies can make an enormous difference in the quality of care you receive from your doctor—and in the quality of care you give yourself. Become more involved in your own health care and see for yourself what a difference it can make in the quality of your life.

ALLERGY HISTORY

• I have experienced the following symptoms (check all those that apply):

___Stuffy or runny nose   ___Postnasal drainage

___Sneezing   ___Itchy or tearing eyes

___Reduction in the sense of taste or smell

___Difficulty getting air into or out of lungs

___Scratchy throat   ___Poor sleep

___Fatigue   ___Frequent need to clear the throat

___Coughing   ___Skin rashes

___Others (list other symptoms: _____)

•When did your symptoms begin? _____

_____

• How often do they occur?

• Do they occur only during certain times of the year?

   ___Spring   ___Summer

   ___Fall   ___Winter

• These symptoms tend to develop or worsen when I spend time:

   ___Indoors   ___At work/school
   ___Outdoors

• My symptoms worsen when I am exposed to:

   ___Outdoor pollen   ___Mold

   ___House dust

   ___Pets (which pets: _____)

• My symptoms worsen in the following specific circumstances (for example, while gardening, raking leaves, taking morning walks, upon waking in the morning, etc.):

• I am taking, or have taken in the past, the following medications (prescription or over-the-counter) to treat my symptoms:

• I am taking the following medications (prescription or over-the-counter) for

other conditions: _____

_____

• List family members that have had allergies: _____

_____

FOLLOW-UP VISIT ALLERGY HISTORY

• Since my last visit, I have experienced the following symptoms

(check all those that apply):

___Stuffy or runny nose ___Postnasal drainage

___Sneezing ___Itchy or tearing eyes

___Reduction in the sense of taste or smell

___Difficulty getting air into or out of lungs

___Scratchy throat ___Poor sleep

___Fatigue ___Frequent need to clear the throat

___Coughing ___Skin rashes

___Others (list other symptoms: _____)

• My symptoms developed or worsened when:

___I spent time indoors ___I spent time outdoors

___I was exposed to pets (which pets: _____)

___I was exposed to mold ___I was exposed to outdoor pollen

___I was exposed to house dust

List all medications you have taken since your last visit. Check off in the *Relief* column those medications that provided effective relief. Also, list any side effects produced by the medication.

Medication	Relief	Side Effects

Resources

The following organizations can provide you with further information about allergies. They may be able to provide you with up-to-date information about recent research and new treatments. In some cases, they may help you locate allergy-related healthcare services in your community.

The Asthma & Allergy Foundation of America (AAFA)
1125 15th Street NW, Suite 502
Washington, DC 20005
(800) 7-ASTHMA
www.aafa.org

AAFA Alabama Chapter
150 Inverness Corners, #307
Birmingham, AL 35242
(205) 408-9077
aafaal@aol.com

AAFA Florida Chapter
11700 N. 58th Street, Suite J
Tampa, FL 33617
(813) 983-0244
www.aafaflorida.org

AAFA Georgia State Chapter
115 Camiff Lake
Milledgeville, GA 31061
(912) 452-7886

AAFA Greater Kansas City Chapter
7905 E. 134th Terrace
Grandview, MO 64030
(816) 966-8164 or (888) 542-8252
aafakc@micro.com or www.aafakc.org

AAFA Maryland Chapter
Chester Building, Suite 321
8600 LaSalle Road
Towson, MD 21286
(410) 321-4710
aafamd@bcpl.net or www.aafa-md.org

AAFA Michigan State Chapter
17520 West 12 Mile Road, Suite 102
Southfield, MI 48076
(248) 557-8050 or (888) 444-0333
aafamich@aol.com

AAFA New England Chapter
220 Boylston Street
Chestnut Hill, MA 02467
(617) 965-7771; aafane@aol.com

AAFA New York State Chapter
910 Charles Street
Fredericksburg, VA 22401
(888) 223-2692; aafany@aol.com

AAFA North Texas Chapter
P.O. Box 270819
Flower Mound, TX 75027
(817) 430-9737 or (888) 932-2232
info@aafa-ntx.org

AAFA Northern California Chapter
3030 Bridgeway, Suite 211
Sausalito, CA 94965
(415) 339-8880; info@aafanoca.org

AAFA Southeast Pennsylvania Chapter
2200 Ben Franklin Parkway, Suite 108 North
Philadelphia, PA 19130
(215) 557-9915; aafasepa@mindspring.com

AAFA Southern California Chapter
5900 Wilshire Boulevard, Suite 2330
Los Angeles, CA 90036
(213) 937-7859 or (800) 624-0044
aafasocal@aol.com
www.aafasocal.com

AAFA St. Louis Chapter
9378 Olive Street Road, Suite 206
St. Louis, MO 63132
(314) 692-2422
aafa@inlink.com

AAFA Washington State Chapter
120 Northgate Plaza, Suite 312
Seattle, WA 98125
(206) 368-2866 or (800) 778-2232
aafawa@aafawa.org
www.aafawa.org

Allergy and Asthma Network/Mothers of Asthmatics, Inc.
2751 Prosperity Avenue, Suite 150
Fairfax, VA 22031
(800) 878-4403 or (703) 641-9595

American Academy of Allergy, Asthma and Immunology
611 E. Wells Street
Milwaukee, WI 53202
(800) 822-2762
www.aaaai.org

American College of Allergy, Asthma and Immunology
85 West Algonquin Road, Suite 550
Arlington Heights, IL 60005
(800) 842-7777
http://allergy.mcg.edu

American Lung Association
1740 Broadway
New York, NY 10019
(212) 315-8700
www.lungusa.org

The Food Allergy Network
10400 Eaton Place, Suite 107
Fairfax, VA 22030-2208
(800) 929-4040
www.foodallergy.org

Latex Allergy Information Service, Inc.
176 Roosevelt Avenue
Torrington, CT 06790
(860) 482-6869
www.latexallergyhelp.com

National Allergy Bureau
(800) 9-POLLEN
www.aaaai.org

National Asthma Education and Prevention Program
National Heart, Lung and Blood Institute
P.O. Box 30105
Bethesda, MD 20824
(301) 251-1222
www.nhlbi.nih.gov

National Institute of Allergy and Infectious Diseases
www.niaid.nih.gov

National Jewish Medical and Research Center
1400 Jackson Street
Denver, CO 80206
Lung Line: (800) 222-LUNG
www.njc.org

Bibliography

Introduction

1. Patterson R, Grammer LC, Greenberger PA (eds.). *Allergic Diseases: Diagnosis and Management. 5th Ed.* Lippincott and Raven. 1997.

2. U.S. Department of Health and Human Services. *Allergic Diseases.* 1991.

Chapter One

1. American Academy of Allergy, Asthma and Immunology. *Allergic Diseases.* 1995.

2. American Academy of Allergy, Asthma and Immunology. *What Is An Allergic Reaction?* 1995.

3. The Asthma and Allergy Foundation of America. *Allergy Basics.* 1995.

4. Creticos PS. Allergic Rhinitis. In: Lichtenstein L, Fauci A (eds.). *Current Therapy in Allergy, Immunology, and Rheumatology.* Mosby. 1996.

5. Fireman P. Allergic Rhinitis. In: Fireman P, Slavin RG (eds.). *Atlas of Allergies.* Mosby-Wolfe. 1996.

6. U.S. Department of Health and Human Services. *Allergic Diseases.* 1991.

Chapter Two

1. American Academy of Allergy, Asthma and Immunology. *Allergic Diseases.* 1995.

2. American Academy of Allergy, Asthma and Immunology. *Allergic Rhinitis, Pollen & Mold Spores.*

3. American Academy of Allergy, Asthma and Immunology. *Pollen and Spores Around the World.* 1996.

4. American Academy of Allergy, Asthma and Immunology. *Understanding the Pollen and Mold Seasons.* 1995.

5. The Asthma and Allergy Foundation of America. *Seasonal Allergies: Pollen and Mold.* 1994.

6. Fireman P, Jelks M. Allergens. In: Fireman P, Slavin RG (eds.). *Atlas of Allergies.* Mosby-Wolfe. 1996.

7. Nacierio R, Solomon W. Rhinitis and Inhalant Allergens. *JAMA.* 278:1842-1848. 1997.

8. National Institute of Allergy and Infectious Diseases. *Something in the Air: Airborne Allergens.* 1993.

Chapter Three

1. American Academy of Allergy, Asthma and Immunology. *Allergies to Animals.* 1995.

2. American Academy of Allergy, Asthma and Immunology. *Dust Mites.* 1995.

3. American Academy of Allergy, Asthma and Immunology. *Removing House Dust and Other Allergic Irritants From Your Home.* 1995.

4. American Academy of Allergy, Asthma and Immunology. *Understanding the Pollen and Mold Seasons.* 1995.

5. The Asthma and Allergy Foundation of America. *Household Allergies: Dust, Mold, Pets, and Cockroaches.* 1994.

6. Bollinger ME, Eggleston PA, et al. Clinical Aspects of Allergic Disease. *Journal of Allergy and Clinical Immunology.* 97:907-14. 1996.

7. Corey JP. Environmental Control of Allergens. *Otolaryngology-Head and Neck Surgery.* 111:340-7. 1994.

8. Creticos PS. Allergic Rhinitis. In: Lichtenstein L, Fauci A (eds.). *Current Therapy in Allergy, Immunology, and Rheumatology.* Mosby. 1996.

9. National Institute of Allergy and Infectious Diseases. *How to Create a Dust-Free Bedroom.* June 1997.

10. National Institute of Allergy and Infectious Diseases. *Something in the Air: Airborne Allergens.* 1993.

11. Van Metre TE. *Cat-Induced Asthma.* The Asthma and Allergy Foundation of America.

Chapter Four

1. The Asthma and Allergy Foundation of America. *Allergy Basics.* 1995.

2. Fireman P. Diagnosis of Allergic Disorders. *Pediatrics in Review.* 16:178-183. 1995.

3. Noble SL, Forbes RC, Woodbridge HB. Allergic Rhinitis. *American Family Physician.* 837-846. 1995.

4. Slavin RG. Diagnostic Tests in Allergy. In: Fireman P, Slavin RG (eds.). *Atlas of Allergies.* Mosby-Wolfe. 1996.

Chapter Five

1. Adelsberg BR. Sedation and Performance Issues in the Treatment of Allergic Conditions. *Archives of Internal Medicine.* 157:494-500. 1997.

2. American Academy of Allergy, Asthma and Immunology. *Allergic Diseases.* 1995.

3. American Pharmaceutical Association. *APhA Special Report: Achieving Optimal Outcomes from Nonprescription Drug Therapy for Allergic Rhinitis.* 1997.

4. Creticos PS. Allergic Rhinitis. In: Lichtenstein L, Fauci A (eds.). *Current Therapy in Allergy, Immunology, and Rheumatology.* Mosby. 1996.

5. Creticos PS. Immunotherapy of Allergic Diseases. In: Lichtenstein L, Fauci A (eds.). *Current Therapy in Allergy, Immunology, and Rheumatology.* Mosby. 1996.

6. Creticos PS. Immunotherapy with Allergens. *JAMA.* 268:2834-2839. 1992.

7. Eleas EF. *Adverse Effects from Asthma and Allergy Medications.* The Asthma and Allergy Foundation of America.

8. Gordon BR. Immunotherapy Basics. *Otolaryngology-Head and Neck Surgery.* 113:597-602. 1995.

9. Kay GG, et al. Initial and Steady-State Effects of Diphenhydramine and Loratadine on Sedation, Cognition, Mood, and Psychomotor Performance. *Archives of International Medicine.* 157:2350-56. 1997.

10. Noble SL, Forbes RC, Woodbridge HB. Allergic Rhinitis. *American Family Physician.* 837-846. 1995.

11. O'Hanlon JF. Antihistamines and Driving Safety. *Cutis.* 42:10-13. 1988.

12. O'Hanlon JF, Ramaekers JG. Antihistamine Effects on Actual Driving Performance in a Standard Test: A Summary of Dutch Experience, 1989-94. *Allergy.* 50:234-242. 1995.

13. Pedinoff AJ. Approaches to the Treatment of Seasonal Allergic Rhinitis. *Southern Medical Journal.* 89:1130-1139. 1996.

14. Philpot E. Allergy Medications: Performance Impairment and Other Issues. *Group Practice Journal.* 65-71. Jan-Feb 1993.

15. Physicians' Online. Beclomethasone Nasal Spray. *Clinical Pharmacology.* 1998.

16. Ricketti, AJ. Allergic Rhinitis. In: Patterson R, Grammer LC, Greenberger PA (eds.). *Allergic Diseases: Diagnosis and Management. 5th Ed.* Lippincott and Raven. 1997.

17. Wright DN, et al. Current Treatment of Allergic Rhinitis and Sinusitis. *Journal of the Florida Medical Association.* 83:391. 1996.

Chapter Six

1. American Academy of Allergy, Asthma and Immunology. *Understanding Food Allergy.* 1993

2. American Academy of Pediatrics. *Allergies in Children.* 1998.

3. American Academy of Pediatrics. *Breastfeeding and the Use of Human Milk.* Policy Statement. December 1997.

4. American Academy of Pediatrics. *Breastfeeding Recommendations* 1997.

5. American Academy of Pediatrics. *Caring for Your Baby and Young Child.* Bantam. 1994.

6. American Academy of Pediatrics. *Starting Solid Foods.* 1997.

7. Bahna SL, Duplantier JE. Food Allergy. *Journal of the Florida Medical Association.* 83:415-418. 1996.

8. Bindslev-Jensen C, Skov PS, Madsen F, Poulsen LK. Food Allergy and Food Intolerance—What is the Difference? *Annals of Allergy.* 72:317-319. 1994.

9. Bock SA. *Food Allergy: A Primer for People.* Vantage Press. 1988.

10. Bock SA, et al. Double-Blind, Placebo-Controlled Food Challenge (DBPCFC) as an Office Procedure: A Manual. *Journal of Allergy and Clinical Immunology.* 82:986-997. 1988.

11. Bush RK, Burks AW, Settipane G. Peanut—A Particularly Powerful and Dangerous Food for Some. *Asthma and Allergy Answers.* The Asthma and Allergy Foundation of America.

12. Clinical Center Communications. National Institutes of Health. *Food Allergy and Intolerances.*

13. Condemi J, Metcalfe DD. Food Allergy in Adults. *Current Therapy in Allergy, Immunology, and Rheumatology* Mosby. 1996.

14. DeSwarte RD. Drug Allergy. In: Patterson R, Grammer LC, Greenberger PA (eds.). *Allergic Diseases: Diagnosis and Management. 5th Ed.* Lippincott and Raven. 1997.

15. Ditto AM, Grammer LC. Food Allergy. In: Patterson R, Grammer LC, Greenberger PA (eds.). *Allergic Diseases: Diagnosis and Management. 5th Ed.* Lippincott and Raven. 1997.

16. Fiocchi A, Restani P, Riva E, Qualizza R, Bruni P, Restelli AR, Galli CL. Meat Allergy: I-Specific IgE to BSA and OSA in Atopic, Beef Sensitive Children. *Journal of the American College of Nutrition.* 14:239-244. 1995.

17. Fireman P. Diagnosis of Allergic Disorders. *Pediatrics in Review.* 16:178-183. 1995.

18. Fireman P. Immunology of Allergic Disorders. *Atlas of Allergies.* Mosby-Wolfe. 1996.

19. Garriga MM, Berkebile C, Metcalfe DD. A Combined Single-Blind, Double-Blind, Placebo-Controlled Study to Determine the Reproducibility of Hypersensitivity Reactions to Aspartame. *Journal of Allergy and Clinical Immunology.* 87:821-7. 1991.

20. Geha R, Buckley CE, Greenberger P, et al. Aspartame is No More Likely Than Placebo to Cause Urticaria/Angioedema: Results of a Multicenter, Randomized, Double-Blind, Placebo-Controlled, Crossover Study. *Journal of Allergy and Clinical Immunology.* 92:513-20. 1993.

21. Goodman DL, McDonnell JT, Nelson HS, et al. Chronic Urticaria Exacerbated by the Antioxidant Food Preservatives, Butylated Hydroxyanisole (BHA) and Butylated Hydroxytoluene (BHT). *Journal of Allergy and Clinical Immunology.* 86:570-5. 1990.

22. Hourihane JO, Dean TP, Warner JO. Peanut Allergy in Relation to Heredity, Maternal Diet, and Other Atopic Diseases: Results of a Questionnaire Survey, Skin Prick Testing, and Food Challenges. *British Medical Journal.* 31:313:518-21. 1996.

23. Kulczycki A. Adverse Reactions to Foods and Food Allergy. In: Korenblat PE, Wedner HJ. *Allergy: Theory and Practice.* W.B. Saunders. 1992.

24. Lehmann P. More Than You Ever Thought You Would Know About Food Additives, Parts I and II. *FDA Consumer.* U.S. Department of Health, Education, and Welfare. 1979.

25. Metcalfe DD. Issues in Diagnosing Food Allergy. *Asthma and Allergy Answers.* The Asthma and Allergy Foundation of America.

26. Munoz-Furlong A. Food Problems: Allergy or Intolerance? *Asthma and Allergy Answers.* The Asthma and Allergy Foundation of America.

27. National Jewish Center for Immunology and Respiratory Medicine. *Understanding Allergy.* 1986.

28. Sampson HA. Diagnosing Food Intolerances in Children. *Current Therapy in Allergy, Immunology, and Rheumatology.* Mosby. 1996.

29. Sampson HA. Food Allergy (Chapter 10). *JAMA.* 278:1888-1894. 1997.

30. Sanker NC. Frazzled by Food Allegies? A Family Odyssey. *Asthma and Allergy Answers.* The Asthma and Allergy Foundation of America.

31. Simon RA. Adverse Reactions to Food Additives. *Asthma and Allergy Answers.* The Asthma and Allergy Foundation of America.

32. Terr AI. Controversial and Unproven Methods in Allergy Diagnosis and Treatment. In: Patterson R, Grammer LC, Greenberger PA (eds.). *Allergic Diseases: Diagnosis and Management. 5th Ed.* Lippincott and Raven. 1997.

33. Teuber SS, Brown RL, Haapanen LAD. Allergenicity of Gourmet Nut Oils Processed by Different Methods. *Journal of Allergy and Clinical Immunology.* 99:502-507. 1997.

34. Watson WTA. Food Allergy in Children. *Clinical Reviews in Allergy and Immunology.* 13:347-359. 1995.

35. Zeiger RS. Preventing Food Allergy in Infants: The Current State of Knowledge. *Asthma and Allergy Answers.* The Asthma and Allergy Foundation of America.

Chapter Seven

1. American Academy of Allergy, Asthma and Immunology. Atopic Dermatitis. *Tips To Remember.*

2. American Academy of Allergy, Asthma and Immunology. Contact Dermatitis. *Tips To Remember.*

3. American Academy of Allergy, Asthma and Immunology. Hives. *Tips To Remember.*

4. American Academy of Pediatrics News Release. *Study Supports Link Between Food Allergy and Atopic Dermatitis.* March 2, 1997.

5. The Asthma and Allergy Foundation of America. Leaflets Three. *Asthma and Allergy Answers.* 1993.

6. Bilbao I, Aguirre A, Vicente JM, Ration JA, Zabala R, Diaz Perez JL. Allergic Contact Dermatitis Due to 5% Doxepin Cream. *Contact Dermatitis.* Oct;35(4):254-5. 1996.

7. Davis MD, McEvoy MT, el-Azhary RA. Topical Psoralen-Ultraviolet A Therapy for Palmoplantar Dermatoses: Experience with 35 Consecutive Patients. *Mayo Clinical Procedures.* 73(5):407-11. 1998.

8. DeLeo VA. Contact Dermatitis. *Current Therapy in Allergy, Immunology, and Rheumatology.* Mosby. 1996.

9. Fireman P. Atopic Dermatitis. *Atlas of Allergies.* Mosby-Wolfe. 1996.

10. Gupta MA, Gupta AK. Chronic Idiopathic Urticaria Associated with Panic Disorder: A Syndrome Responsive to Selective Serotonin Reuptake Inhibitor Antidepressants? *Cutis.* Jul;56(1):53-4. 1995.

11. Henry Ford Health System (Division of Allergy and Clinical Immunology) and The Asthma and Allergy Foundation of America. *The ABCs of Latex Allergy.* 1997.

12. Kulczycki A, Atkinson JP. Urticaria and Angioedema. In: Korenblat PE, Wedner HJ. *Allergy: Theory and Practice.* W.B. Saunders. 1992.

13. Leung DYM, et al. Allergic and Immunologic Skin Disorders. *JAMA.* 278:1914-1923. 1997.

14. Lawlor F, Greaves MW. Chronic Urticaria. *Current Therapy in Allergy, Immunology, and Rheumatology.* Mosby. 1996.

15. Metzger WJ. Urticaria, Angioedema, and Hereditary Angioedema. In: Patterson R, Grammer LC, Greenberger PA (eds.). *Allergic Diseases: Diagnosis and Management. 5th Ed.* Lippincott and Raven. 1997.

16. Morison WL. Recent Advances in Phototherapy and Photo-chemotherapy of Skin Disease. *Journal of Dermatological Science.* 1(3):141-7. 1990.

17. O'Byrne P, et al. Exercise-Induced Bronchoconstriction, Anaphylaxis, and Urticaria. In: Lichtenstein L, Fauci A (eds.). *Current Therapy in Allergy, Immunology, and Rheumatology.* Mosby. 1996.

18. Ownby DR. Latex Allergy: The Sting of Rubber. *Asthma and Allergy Answers.* The Asthma and Allergy Foundation of America.

19. Paller AS. Atopic Dermatitis. *Current Therapy in Allergy, Immunology, and Rheumatology.* Mosby. 1996.

20. Sabroe RA, Kennedy CT, Archer CB. The Effects of Topical Doxepin on Responses to Histamine, Substance P and Prostaglandin E2 in Human Skin. *British Journal of Dermatology.* Sep;137(3):386-90. 1997.

21. Slavin RG. Allergic Contact Dermatitis. *Atlas of Allergies.* Mosby-Wolfe. 1996.

22. Soter NA. Physical Urticaria-Angioedema. *Current Therapy in Allergy, Immunology, and Rheumatology.* Mosby. 1996.

23. Tharp MD, Levine MI, Fireman P. Urticaria and Angioedema. *Atlas of Allergies.* Mosby-Wolfe. 1996.

24. Ylitalo L, et al. Natural Rubber Latex Allergy in Children Who Had Not Undergone Surgery and Children Who Had Undergone Multiple Operations. *Journal of Allergy and Clinical Immunology.* 100:5; 606-612. November 1997.

Chapter Eight

1. Brockow K, Kiehn M, Riethmuller C, Vieluf D, Berger J, Ring J. Efficacy of Antihistamine Pretreatment in the Prevention of Adverse Reactions to Hymenoptera Immunotherapy: A Prospective, Randomized, Placebo-Controlled Trial. *Journal of Allergy and Clinical Immunology.* Oct;100(4):458-63. 1997.

2. Golden DB. Allergic Reactions to Insect Stings. In: Middleton E, Reed CE, Elliot E (eds.). *Allergy: Principles and Practice. 4th Ed.* Mosby Year Book. 1993.

3. Graft DF. Insect Sting Allergy in Adults. *Current Therapy in Allergy, Immunology, and Rheumatology.* Mosby. 1996.

4. *Physicians' Desk Reference. 52nd Edition.* Medical Economics Company. 1998.

5. Reisman RE. Allergy to Stinging Insects. In: Patterson R, Grammer LC, Greenberger PA (eds.). *Allergic Diseases: Diagnosis and Management. 5th Ed.* Lippincott and Raven. 1997.

Chapter Nine

1. DeShazo RD, Kemp SF. Allergic Reactions to Drugs and Biologic Agents. *JAMA.* 278:1895-1906. 1997.

2. DeShazo RD, Smith DL. Drug Reactions. *Current Therapy in Allergy, Immunology, and Rheumatology.* Mosby. 1996.

3. DeSwarte RD. Drug Allergy. In: Patterson R, Grammer LC, Greenberger PA (eds.). *Allergic Diseases: Diagnosis and Management. 5th Ed.* Lippincott and Raven. 1997.

4. Fireman P. Atopic Dermatitis. *Atlas of Allergies.* Mosby-Wolfe. 1996.

5. Grammer LC. Drug Allergy. *Atlas of Allergies.* Mosby-Wolfe. 1996.

6. Kaplan MS. Penicillin Allergy. *Current Therapy in Allergy, Immunology, and Rheumatology.* Mosby. 1996.

7. *Physicians' Desk Reference. 52nd Edition.* Medical Economics Company. 1998.

8. Roujeau JC. Stevens-Johnson Syndrome and Toxic Epidermal Necrolysis are Severity Variants of the Same Disease Which Differs from Erythema Multiforme. *Journal of Dermatology.* Nov;24(11):726-9. 1997.

9. Slavin RG. Allergic Contact Dermatitis. *Atlas of Allergies.* Mosby-Wolfe. 1996.

10. Tharp MD, Levine MI, Fireman P. Urticaria and Angioedema. *Atlas of Allergies.* Mosby-Wolfe. 1996.

11. VanArsdel PP. Drug Hypersensitivity. In: Middleton E, Reed CE, Elliot E (eds.). *Allergy: Principles and Practice. 4th Ed.* Mosby Year Book. 1993.

Chapter Ten

1. Aeling JL. Contact Dermatitis. In: Middleton E, Reed CE, Elliot E (eds.). *Allergy: Principles and Practice. 4th Ed.* Mosby Year Book. 1993.

2. American Academy of Allergy, Asthma and Immunology. *Allergic Contact Dermatitis.* 1998.

3. Bernstein DI. Allergic Reactions to Workplace Allergens. *JAMA.* 278:1907-1913. 1997.

4. Bernstein JA, Bernstein DI, Bernstein IL. Occupational Asthma. In: Middleton E, Reed CE, Elliot E (eds.). *Allergy: Principles and Practice. 4th Ed.* Mosby Year Book. 1993.

5. Chan-Yeung MC, Malo JL. Aetiologic Agents in Occupational Asthma. *European Respiratory Journal.* 7:346-371. 1994.

6. Chan-Yeung MC, Malo JL. Occupational Asthma. *New England Journal of Medicine.* 333:107-111. 1995.

7. Cullen M. Multiple Chemical Sensitivities. In: Last JM, Wallace RB (eds.). *Public Health and Preventive Medicine.* Appleton and Lang. 1992.

8. DeLeo VA. Contact Dermatitis. *Current Therapy in Allergy, Immunology, and Rheumatology.* Mosby. 1996.

9. Fischman ML. Building Associated Illness. In: LaDou J. *Occupational Medicine.* Appleton and Lang. 1990.

10. Henry Ford Health System (Division of Allergy and Clinical Immunology) and The Asthma and Allergy Foundation of America. *The ABCs of Latex Allergy.* 1997.

11. Morren MA, Janssens V, Dooms-Gossens A, Van Hoeyveld E, Cornelis A, De Wolf-Peeters C, Heremans A. Alpha-Amylase, a Flour Additive: An Important Cause of Protein Contact Dermatitis in Bakers. *Journal of the American Academy of Dermatology.* Nov;29(5 Pt 1):723-8. 1993.

12. Occupational Immunologic Lung Disease. In: Patterson R, Grammer LC, Greenberger PA (eds.). *Allergic Diseases: Diagnosis and Management. 5th Ed.* Lippincott and Raven. 1997.

13. Revsbech P, Dueholm M. Storage Mite Allergy Among Bakers. *Allergy.* Apr;45(3):204-8. 1990.

14. Slavin RG. Allergic Contact Dermatitis. In: Patterson R, Grammer LC, Greenberger PA (eds.). *Allergic Diseases: Diagnosis and Management. 5th Ed.* Lippincott and Raven. 1997.

15. Slavin RG. Occupational Allergies. In: Fireman P, Slavin RG. (eds.). *Atlas of Allergies.* Mosby-Wolfe. 1996.

16. Valdivieso R, Subiza J, Subiza JL, Hinojosa M, de Carlos E, Subiza E. Bakers' Asthma Caused by Alpha Amylase. *Annals of Allergy.* Oct;73(4):337-42. 1994.

17. Veach M. Latex Gloves Hand Health Workers A Growing Worry. *American Medical News.* Vol. 40, Number 38. 1997.

Chapter Eleven

1. American Academy of Allergy, Asthma and Immunology. *Triggers of Asthma.* 1995.

2. The Asthma and Allergy Foundation of America. *A Report on the Revised Guidelines for the Diagnosis and Management of Asthma.* Summer 1997.

3. The Asthma and Allergy Foundation of America. *Asthma Basics.* 1994.

4. Corren J. Allergic Rhinitis and Asthma: How Important Is the Link? *Journal of Allergy and Clinical Immunology.* 99:S781-S786. 1997.

5. Creticos PS. Asthma in Adults. In: Lichtenstein L, Fauci A (eds.). *Current Therapy in Allergy, Immunology, and Rheumatology.* Mosby. 1996.

6. Greenberger PA. Asthma. In: Patterson R, Grammer LC, Greenberger PA (eds.). *Allergic Diseases: Diagnosis and Management. 5th Ed.* Lippincott and Raven. 1997.

7. Kaliner M, Lemanske R. Rhinitis and Asthma. *JAMA.* 268:2807-2829. 1992.

8. Lemanske RF, Busse WW. Asthma. *JAMA.* 278:1855-1880. 1997.

9. National Jewish Center for Immunology and Respiratory Medicine. *Your Child and Asthma.* 1992.

10. *Physicians' Desk Reference. 52nd Edition.* Medical Economics Company. 1998.

11. Skoner DP. Asthma. *Atlas of Allergies.* Mosby-Wolfe. 1996.

12. Small RE, Kennedy DT. New Asthma Guidelines: Applications for Pharmaceutical Care. *Journal of the American Pharmaceutical Association.* NS37:419-437. 1997.

13. U.S. Department of Health & Human Services. *Allergic Diseases.* 1991.

14. Utell MJ, Looney RJ. Environmentally Induced Asthma. *Toxicology Letters.* 82:47-53. 1995.

Chapter Twelve

1. National Jewish Center for Immunology and Respiratory Medicine. *Your Child and Asthma.* 1992.

2. U.S. Department of Health and Human Services. *Allergic Diseases.* 1991.

Index